Searching Young Hearts

Searching Young Hearts
Adolescent Sexuality and Spirituality

Robert Doolittle

Saint Mary's Press
Christian Brothers Publications
Winona, Minnesota

This book is dedicated to Paul Sullivan and Paul Cain,
in gratitude for their years of faithful trust building with the youth
of Saint Agnes.

Nihil Obstat: Rev. Jerome E. Listecki
Censor Deputatus
29 September 1993
Imprimatur: †Most Rev. John G. Vlazny, DD
Bishop of Winona
29 September 1993

The publishing team included Robert P. Stamschror, development editor; Rebecca L. Fairbank, manuscript editor; Amy Schlumpf Manion, typesetter; Michael and Suzanne Welch/Studio Sphere, cover designers; Evy Abrahamson, illustrator; pre-press, printing, and binding by the graphics division of Saint Mary's Press.

Contents

Introduction

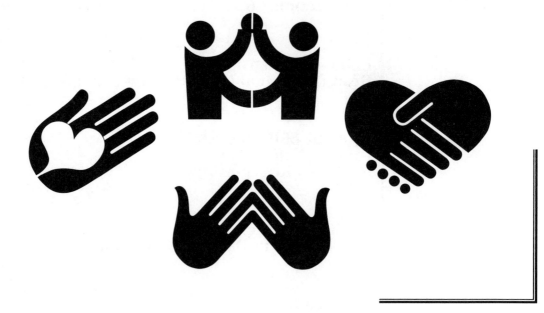

Searching Young Hearts

In *Searching Young Hearts,* you will find plans for building a sturdy bridge of trust on which you can cross the chasm of silence that separates most of our young people from adult help in dealing with sexuality in their lives and relationships.

Young people need to talk about their sexuality, and they need us present as listeners, but these needs usually go unmet. Young people also need coaching from us, and we frequently ache with things we would like to say, if only we could.

We look awkwardly at one another across a silence we do not know how to break. The young people fear, perhaps, that they will look sappy and immature if they ask, and we fear that we will sound moralistic and old-fashioned if we speak.

We need bridges to cross that fearful silence. And thanks to the bridge-building work of many candid teens and adults at Saint Agnes Parish in Reading, Massachusetts, where I was privileged to minister as youth coordinator, I am able to offer in this book a series of sturdy and well-tested bridges to break that silence.

In the pages that follow, I not only give you the programs we invented to open up dialog, but I also invite you to see and to feel the actual struggles of both generations who took the risk of communicating and growing together.

In offering our programs on sexuality, I am really passing on to you, as a person who ministers to young people, a challenge from the teens and adults of Saint Agnes Parish. We are challenging you to struggle and grow, like we did, in a sensitive area where love and faith, sex and conscience, and God and self all meet. The issues waiting to be discussed are heavy with heartfelt meaning and deeply contested values, yet they are also light due to the hopes and the ready laughter of youth.

Please, please do not approach young people just to "straighten out their twisted morals." That approach is itself twisted and condescending. "Papa Don't Preach," the title of a song by Madonna, is a cry with which every young heart resonates. Go to them to ask and to listen. Go to tell them your own personal story of search, struggle, and discovery. Go with a love for them that is greater than your love for the heartfelt values you have to share. Do share those values with all your heart, but share them as part of a larger love that moves you and the young people to undertake the shared risk of opening yourselves to one another and of coming to know one another deeply.

For teenagers, the issue of sex is primarily an issue of intimacy—the want of intimacy, the power of intimacy, the lack of intimacy. So let all the sessions you develop from this book be intimate sessions in which both generations are invited to be open—with stories, laughter, tears, passionate convictions, scary confusions, old hurts, new hopes, and tough decisions. If we are to improve young people's understanding of love, the sessions themselves need to be experiences of great love—feasts of warmth, trust, and close feelings. Let the message of Christ and the wisdom of the church pour in through listening, sharing, understanding, and affirming, not just through presenting a list of black-and-white do's and don'ts that may drive a lot of teens off in the wrong direction.

And yes, many young people are going in the wrong direction—a crazy, self-damaging direction. According to a public opinion poll for Planned Parenthood, more than 50 percent of teens in the United States are sexually active, and there's no reason to think Catholic teens are exempt from that statistic (Faye Wattleton, "American Teens: Sexually Active, Sexually Illiterate," *Education Digest* [March 1988]: 51). Maybe that fact puts you off. Maybe it scares you. Maybe it disgusts you and offends your sense of decency. Let me propose another response—deep compassion. Yes, many young people are treating their bodies and their futures carelessly, partying too much and getting in way over their heads with sex. But they are still teens, and they are still searching for what is right, even as they try out values and behaviors that put them at risk.

Underneath their masks of self-assurance, young people are still trying to figure out what road leads to happiness and fulfillment. And that means there is still a place and a need in their lives for you and me. A silent cry from that carefully guarded wondering of theirs calls to us.

How to Use *Searching Young Hearts*

I have two practical suggestions for using this book. The first comes from Lee Selzer, a former youth group member, now a parish youth coordinator. Lee suggests using this book not as a resource for the expected annual "sex and love" session, but rather using this material—there's enough here—to keep the subject alive all year long, maybe once a month or so. That way the shared thinking that takes place in group sessions can keep pace with the private thinking that the young people do in exploring their own emerging sexuality.

The second suggestion is from me. The programs in this book were all developed with and for high school young people during the 1980s. But now by the time most teens reach high school, they have all but completed their work on sex values. They will still greatly benefit if we open up a dialog of trust with them, and they will appreciate this dialog, even though it will be increasingly difficult for them. Therefore, I strongly recommend that much of this material be introduced at the eighth-, seventh-, and even sixth-grade levels. That is when the values are being formed, so that is when we need to be there for the young people.

Reproducing Handouts

To preserve the binding of this book, first reproduce a master copy of the pages to be handed out and then use the master copy for future reproductions.

My Prayer for You

I am filled with warm and hopeful feelings for this book, and I pray that in it you will find much courage and feel much attraction for its trust-building work. Our young people *are* a generation at risk. They face all the risks we faced plus risks we never imagined. And it is not an exaggeration to say that they need us to reach out and help them to safety.

1

Hello, Young Lovers: Healthy Spiritual Lives, Healthy Love Lives

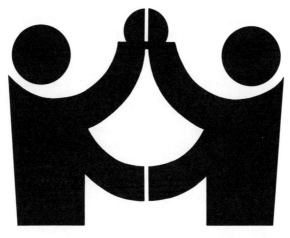

Young people often keep their love lives and their spiritual lives in separate compartments. This inner division is a big mistake. It locks the wisdom of the church and the young people's relationship with Christ—essential parts of themselves—out of their love lives, which normally involve much joy, as well as much confusion and pain.

The Need for Catechesis About Love

Adolescents have a double need concerning love relationships. They need clarity about the realities of love relationships, and they need inner healing from the real hurts love relationships often include. But most often, the catechesis must come first. An eleventh grader named Elaine made me vividly aware of the necessity for that sequence. While confiding in me about her stormy love situation, she was startled when I suggested there was a spiritual issue involved. She responded: "Bob, don't get religious on me. This is real-life stuff I'm going through." The compartments of her love life and her spiritual life were perfectly sealed off. Only months later, when she was part of a large-group discussion on romantic love, could Elaine break through the wall between her love life and her spirituality and ask for prayer to help heal a love attachment that had eroded her inner stability. The catechesis imparted in the group discussion about romantic love equipped her with the perspective she needed to name her problem.

Elaine's pain at the group session was the same pain she had been dealing with when we had first talked, but in the group discussion she got hold of a few principles of healthy love relationships and could see how violations of those principles were causing her pain. She could then ask for help to mend the broken place in her heart, because she could finally see the unhealthy patterns she had developed.

Our teens need us to name, for them and with them, the spiritual wisdom we have gained about the love problems they face. Until we do, it simply never occurs to most of them that Christ and the church have much to offer their love lives. Once that realization dawns, the young people often find that they already have spiritual wisdom that applies quite appropriately to the love-life decisions they have to make. The naming and clarifying of love relationship realities, which precedes and makes possible later healing of young people's love hurts, is the purpose of the catechesis in this chapter.

Opening the Catechetical Door

How can we open the door to the young people's "love compartments" and let in the light of Gospel catechesis? On what grounds can we bring up such a sensitive and private subject as this? Two keys will help to open the door.

The first key is to affirm the young people's romantic quest as an important and legitimate part of their personal learning agenda. Silence about love-life issues may give the young people the impression that we consider the ups and downs of young love to be trivial. We must convince them that their romantic concerns are so important to us that we want them to acquire the spiritual perspectives and resources they will need to deal with all the pitfalls they will face in their love lives. Only then will their struggling, searching young hearts be open to the spiritual formation and healing we offer. If their experience has been that church people have had only a negative interest in their love lives, we can admit that this may have been true. But we can also say that the church and we as church representatives now have a new concern and a fresh, positive approach. And we can promise that this approach will be of great help to them by enabling love to happen in a healthy and happy way.

The second key is an honest boldness about love and sex. We can be frank about wanting them to come of age with healthy love responses to one another. And we can propose that healthy love responses require a clear grasp of what love is all about. We can add that at the present time, our society doesn't offer much clarity on the subject, but a Christian perspective does.

If we use affirmation and honesty urgently and gently, few youth groups will be able to resist—even if only for curiosity's sake—wanting to know what on earth the church does have to offer them.

Building the Mood for Catechesis on Sex and Love

A mood of personal openness to catechesis on sex and love can be effective. To illustrate, I will describe the events, the thinking, and the preparation that took place before a memorable meeting we had with our young people on premarital sex.

To my knowledge, over a fifteen-year period, five female members of our parish youth group had become pregnant—two before they graduated, three not long afterward. All five had their babies—one chose adoption, the other four chose single parenthood. All five earned the respect of people around them for the way they handled the sudden adult decision they faced.

I still have warm—and even proud—feelings for each of those young women. However, each of their pregnancies hit me hard. They indicated to me that we had failed to hand on to those teens, persuasively enough, the Gospel values about sexuality.

After the last of those young women had her baby we knew we had to do a lot more to help our teens buck the culture and abstain from sex until marriage. But what could we do?

Many fine films and programs advocating abstinence from sex before marriage were available. However, we knew that no media blitz, however polished, could undo the years of media conditioning that had most teens in a mindless daze about sex.

We believed the necessary waker-upper to the pitfalls of young love would be a wide-open discussion of what is helpful and what is harmful in teen love relationships. I say a "discussion," because we recognized that even a beautifully candid and caring speech by an admired adult would still not change young hearts. Those hearts needed an opportunity to open up and hold out their searching questions, their honest opinions, their painful experiences, and their deep concerns. Teens would not be likely to open up in response to a lecture, which was the standard approach a generation or two ago. But perhaps they would open up if we were willing to "hear where they're at," respect their dignity as decision-makers, and respond with loving candor to ideas that could hurt them.

That was our hope. What we undertook, then, was not so much an effort to persuade as it was a leap into mutual truthfulness about sex and love. In taking this approach, we were aware of a plain truth that we as adults simply had to accept: *We are talking with young adults who have young adult bodies and young adult wills, and we the older adult church, whether as parents or as teachers, cannot control what they will do.*

To try to manipulate young people's wills would be to take on the character of a cult. Cults attempt to control the thinking and the decision-making of their disciples. They bury the free and responsible human person. Better an untimely pregnancy than that. Especially with teenagers—where a responsible launching into adulthood was at stake—our mission had to be aimed at larger thinking, better decision-making, and greater, not less, responsibility of the person. With that approach, there would be a better chance that the young people would welcome us and our urgent topic, feeling, "Here at last is someone who knows I'm not a child, yet knows I need company and intelligent conversation to help me in exploring my sexuality."

Representing this approach, I met with our peer leadership group, and we searched for a mood-setting starting point that would foster helpful discussion on sexuality. The group proposed establishing an initial ground rule for the whole group. Ground rules do not usually open young people's hearts, but this one did. The ground rule was this: "About sex, people will disagree—strongly! And it is very easy to slip into disrespect for those who disagree with us. With this topic, we touch one another's most sensitive hopes and feelings. Nothing less than profound mutual respect will do. And along with that respect must be an equally profound willingness to disagree lovingly."

When that ground rule was announced on the night of our much-anticipated meeting, a holy hush—I do not exaggerate—swept through the room. We all knew the session would be good, and it was.

To our amazement, people shared the anguish that their parents', and even their grandparents', sexual irresponsibilities had caused them. No one debated at all that night. Instead we heard what it was like when young people compared birth dates and wedding dates and realized that they had been conceived out of wedlock. Some shed quiet tears. Others shared stories about friends their age with babies and lost opportunities to finish growing up. As a leadership team, we had accomplished our goal by creating that open group mood. No coaching about abstinence from premarital sex was needed from adults that night. The realities of irresponsible sex just rose from people's hearts, where they had been locked away, and any misconceptions about those realities were just blown away, almost effortlessly.

Seven Sessions on Love for Young Lovers

The rest of this chapter presents seven sessions for exploring with the young people seven aspects of their love lives. Each session draws from and is supported by a scriptural passage. The sessions are designed to be both interesting and empowering to all the young lovers you hope to help.

Session Content and Underlying Values

The catechetical content for each session is presented to you, the leader, in the form of a short piece of practical advice for love-coaching young people. These love-coaching resources are placed on separate pages at the end of the chapter so that you may photocopy them if you wish. Although they are directed to you, the resources can become catechetical content for the young people by giving them copies and letting them read them critically. You can tell them to read these pieces as if they are eavesdropping on a conversation among adults about the sexuality of young people. (The piece for session 7 is an exception. It is a letter addressed directly to the young people.)

Two primary values are contained in each of the seven love-coaching resources: One is wholeness of person, and the other is keenness of conscience.

The value of wholeness of person is communicated by helping the young people see that becoming spiritually whole means becoming humanly and sexually whole. Attracting, welcoming, and genuinely responding to the other sex and to their own emerging maleness or femaleness are all parts of that wholeness.

The value of keenness of conscience is communicated by helping the young people become thoughtful and prayerful about the way they treat the sacred trust of a love involvement. The sessions encourage the young people to welcome and never stifle the prompting of the Spirit in the love decisions they make.

With these twin values in mind, the words of Jesus come through with new resonance, "'Thy faith hath made thee whole'" (Matt. 9:22, KJV). In the context of helping young people address their love concerns, this passage translates into "your prayer life can do great things for your love life."

Session Method

- To help the young people engage actively in their reading of the love-coaching resources, tell them to underline anything that evokes a response and code it in the margin. Ask them to make a plus sign (+) beside any point they really like, a minus sign (-) beside any point they take issue with, and a question mark (?) beside any point they don't understand.
- Start each discussion by asking the group members to take turns sharing one item they marked and why. After everyone has shared, let the discussion take its own course.
- As a final discussion question, refer the group to the Gospel passage or passages in each of the love-coaching resources and ask the group members what they hear Jesus saying to them about the situation explored in that piece.

For each of the love-coaching resources, I have included a commentary to help you use the advice to its fullest potential.

Session 1

The Two Faces of Love

I have written this introductory session to the serious subjects of spirituality and sexuality in a serious fashion. But there is no need to present the material that way. The love-coaching advice, just by its subject matter, will surely rivet the attention of your young readers. You might extend the atmosphere of openness by introducing a note of playfulness. Perhaps a remark like this will start up their humor motors: "But sex is too sensitive for us to discuss, and after all, this is church! What? Do I detect some interest here?" Then you will have a green light to do some serious learning together. (See "Love-Coaching Resource for Session 1" on page 17.)

Session 2

The Idol of Love

The session 2 advice is extremely countercultural. It undercuts the sentimental premise of most movies, songs, soap operas, and stories. The discussion can evoke a judgmental arrogance in some, and it will surely challenge the deep longings of others. The discussion leader should insist on compassion rather than cynicism toward the tendency in all of us to fall into the tender trap of the goddess Venus and her imp, Cupid.

Your group members may quickly grasp why it is dangerous to worship romantic love or any other sort of idol. Or they may need to explore other examples and see that all idols exercise a certain appeal, but that none can deliver the way Christ does. (See "Love-Coaching Resource for Session 2" on page 18.)

Session 3   ### True Friendship

Session 3 uses the highly charged word *friendship* to bridge the separation between the consciences and love patterns of the young people. You will not have to tell them how they should be treating each other. Your job is simply to keep the questions in sharp focus so that the conscience-considered answers about friendship that the young people already know can better connect these two often unconnected areas of their lives. (See "Love-Coaching Resource for Session 3" on page 19.)

Session 4   ### Praying Together

Okay, youth leader, consider yourself challenged. Try praying with someone you love. That will allow you to speak firsthand about the benefits and the difficulties entailed in opening up a love relationship to Christ. Help your group members realize how ready Christ is to enter and assist in any area of their lives, but only if he is invited. (See "Love-Coaching Resource for Session 4" on page 20.)

Session 5   ### Breaking Up

Your purpose in session 5 is to help your young people trust the ending of relationships as much as their beginning. Perhaps your group will be able to see here the deep truth of life, death, and resurrection that is the dynamic of the Eucharist and of all human growth. (See "Love-Coaching Resource for Session 5" on page 21.)

Session 6   ### An Open Letter to Magic Johnson

A few weeks after Magic Johnson spoke on the "Arsenio Hall Show," advocating the use of condoms for safe sex, he made a different pitch: "No sex is the only real safe sex." However, his later pitch got a lot less press coverage in most areas than his first effort, and even if his later pitch had been given equal coverage, it wouldn't have come close to the exposure that Arsenio Hall has among young people. So the damage was already done.

The point of this session is not just the condom issue. If your young people accept the logic of this open letter, their voices can live its values and spread its message. Their "light" is necessary. The voices of young people in Cambridge, Massachusetts, pushed condom distribution into place in their high school. Young people can likewise raise their voices in favor of abstinence and have a big influence on what takes place. (See "Love-Coaching Resource for Session 6" on page 22.)

Session 7

What Sex Does for and Against Love

I strongly recommend asking some parishioners to get together and pray in support of this session. The young people will probably not agree with this session's advice, but a vigorous discussion is guaranteed. The power of the church's urgent warnings will have a positive effect, regardless of whether people accept them on the spot. Your job is to clearly present the Gospel values and the reasons for them. Then the young people will make their own choices in light of that information and those values. (See "Love-Coaching Resource for Session 7" on pages 23–25.)

The Two Faces of Love

> "I am telling you not to worry about your life . . . or about your body and what you are to wear. . . . Your heavenly Father knows you need them all. Set your hearts on his kingdom first, . . . and all these other things will be given you as well." (Matthew 6:25,32–33, NJB)

Love is supposed to be so great and wonderful, but think for a minute about how badly people in love sometimes hurt each other. We have to ask, "Why can't love live up to its name?"

Perhaps knowing that love has two faces can help answer that question. The word *love* can have two different meanings, and the Greek language actually uses two separate words. *Eros* means romantic love, which is about attraction, and *agape* means generous love, which is about caring and true friendship. Much of the pain in our love life happens because the romantic, attracting sort of love, eros, is pursued without caring, without real friendship, or agape. When this is the case, we run over each other in the pursuit of our own happiness. But love between the sexes does not have to be like that. People can treat each other gently and generously. Eros and agape are different, but they need not be at odds.

And that brings us to the word and the reality we are dealing with: *sexuality*. Sexuality is masculinity or femininity—the male style in response to others, especially females, and the female style in response to others, especially males. Now here is an astounding fact: Eros—romance and attraction—as it emerges in a young person's masculinity or femininity, actually blossoms more fully if agape—generosity and real friendship—leads the way. What? Do I really mean to say that good-heartedness confers a cosmetic advantage, that generosity enhances romance and attractiveness?

Jesus puts it this way: "'Your heavenly Father knows [all your needs]. But seek first the kingdom [of God] . . . and all these things will be given you besides'" (Matthew 6:32–34, NAB). God knows that young people have a great need to grow in attractiveness. However, this healthy goal can sometimes become a consuming obsession—a driven kind of selfishness. Can we put the Kingdom first, even ahead of our need to be a winner in romance, and then see that need be met more fully as a result? Well, listen to this bit of scriptural wisdom: "The fruit of the Spirit is love, joy, and peace" (Galatians 5:22, NIV). In practical terms, that means the relaxed and caring attitude of a person of God—one who practices agape and gives equal importance to self and others—is beautiful to behold. People of God radiate an appealing strength, warmth, and confidence, all of which show on their face. And male or female attractiveness, or sexuality, is brought out more fully.

The Idol of Love

"'Worship the Lord your God,
and serve only him.'"
(Matthew 4:10, NRSV)

For many young people, the longing to find that one special someone is their deepest hope. Who can blame them? Our culture has taught all of us to place our hopes for happiness, self-worth, and meaning on one bet—romantic love. Unfortunately, that bet is always lost. Having a wonderful boyfriend or girlfriend can never fulfill all our hopes.

Our culture's call to romantic love is an invitation to idolatry. Idolatry is a soul-crushing sin that few teens have ever heard about. Moses made it the first of the Ten Commandments: "'I, the LORD, am your God. . . . You shall not have other gods besides me'" (Exodus 20:2–3, NAB). Idolatry is placing something, like money, or someone, like a girlfriend, ahead of God as the object of one's greatest trust, hope, and desire.

What is so wrong with wanting to be attractive so that we can grab someone and hang on for dear life? That desire is wrong because it becomes an addiction, a form of slavery. That kind of love cannot answer the deep need of our soul to be loved completely and never to be let down. Only Christ can set us free, make us happy, and never fail us. Love songs tell lovely lies when they promise us that much. Those who rest their ultimate hopes on the high and wonderful feelings of romantic love are committing the great self-destructive sin of idolatry and are heading for tremendous disillusionment.

On the other hand, those who keep romantic love in perspective and reserve the heart's total trust for Christ approach romantic love relationships in a very different way. The love feelings that accompany romantic attraction still come powerfully, but not desperately. There is an ability to love generously, but not graspingly. There is still a capacity to feel tremendous joy or sadness as relationships soar or fall, but also an ability and a freedom to have or not have a relationship—and to trust Christ's lead either way. Most of all, there is an ability to let the passionate inner purpose of one's life unfold, which it cannot do when one's whole self is consumed in one other person.

True Friendship

"Love one another as I have loved you. . . . You are my friends if you do what I command you." (John 15:12–14, NRSV)

For teens, *friendship* is a sacred word, a sacred value. This word calls forth the best in them, their highest sense of what one person can be to another. Thus, the standards of friendship can be used to measure real love—before, during, and after becoming involved romantically. "Do to a love partner only what you would do to a good friend" becomes a standard young people can readily use to guide their love decisions. For instance: "Don't get romantically involved until you are friends." "Keep working at a better and better friendship." "Be friends even after the romantic attraction has faded."

But what is friendship? A lot of candid discussion is necessary in this session. We can say openly that romantic love's needs, fears, and selfishness can cramp and twist the flow of friendship between young hearts. Couples often play games of competition, manipulation, concealment, and deception. This jockeying for advantage comes quite naturally when one's own happiness is love's main purpose. Friendship is not selfishness, game playing, or gaining advantage over others. The higher purpose of friendship confronts all those. But we still need to define what friendship

is. Well, friendship is generosity instead of self-centeredness, reconciliation instead of resentment, affirmation instead of put-downs.

And friendship is still more. True friends long to hear the truth of each other's deepest self. The effort to speak and to listen to each other's truest thoughts and feelings is the essential business of friendship. Thus, friendship is the practice of truth, of seeking the person within.

So friends are truth-seekers and truth-tellers. But let's be honest: It is hard to open up. Is it worth the price? To take up the challenge of openness and honesty is to declare friendship to the inner self of one's friend and to invite that person to come out fully. That is an incredible gift to give. Is it worth it? Definitely!

When wielding the word *friendship*, young people can do great things. Now agape can critique eros and keep it healthy. Now dating partners can become a source of blessing instead of anguish to each other. Now partners with abusive tendencies can be challenged to change. And now mutual concern, honesty, and growth can become the mission of our teens as they set out to love.

Praying Together

> "Where two or three are gathered together in my name, there
> am I in the midst of them." (Matthew 18:20, NAB)

If a couple in love want to seek true friendship, another level of trust can be opened to put the relationship on an even more solid footing.

The idea of two people turning to Christ together in prayer is really quite simple. However, a love relationship is usually an exclusive and closed world between two people. For that reason, what I am proposing may at first seem quite strange to most teens, and even to most adults. But if one partner in a relationship has just been hit with a painful loss of some sort, what could be more natural than for the other partner to offer a short prayer of comfort? And if a couple are faced with a big decision, what could be more practical than to pray together, "God help us"? Or perhaps they are faced with an argument, event, or project.

I suggest taking hands occasionally and talking to Christ together—honestly speaking from the heart in each other's presence. Praying together is a simple way to let Christ into a relationship, and the blessings that follow are enormous.

Actually, the practice of couples praying together, even when dating, can be a foundation for future family prayer among Catholics. I propose that young unmarried couples pray together, because I firmly believe that shared spirituality is the foundation of a healthy marriage and family. I also propose that the teen years are the right time for such experimentation because these are the years for building up the repertoire of relational skills that young people will later bring to marriage.

Resource 1–D: Permission to reproduce this resource is granted.

Breaking Up

"Unless a grain of wheat falls into the earth and dies, it
remains just a single grain; but if it dies, it bears much fruit."
(John 12:24, NRSV)

Dean Borgman of the Center for Youth Studies at Gordon Conwell Seminary in Wenham, Massachusetts, once said that teens can expect to have about three important love relationships before meeting their marriage partner. That could mean going through three crushing, confidence-blowing breakups. Or is there a better way?

Try out this strange-sounding advice on young people:

Going with someone is good, and so is breaking up. In fact, going with and breaking up with several someones is a good thing. Each relationship can offer something of value to the growth of both partners. Once that growth is complete, the fire goes out, and it's simply time to move on. This moving on is not at all a failure; it's a normal, healthy step—good for the individual and good preparation for marriage.

The permanent possession in relationships is not each other. Rather, it is the growing you do together. So when the time to break up comes, be ready for it. Shed some tears for the good relationship you had, give each other a great big thank you, and part as warm friends.

There is one more thing: If you want a relationship to end on good terms, do not have sex. Lovemaking awakens the need for permanency. That need is natural and powerful. Consequently, the breakup of a sexually active relationship leaves wounds far more painful and long-term than a normal breakup.

After our youth group discussed that advice, several couples in the group were able to break up when the time came, stay friends, and remain in the group—instead of one of them leaving the youth group, which sometimes happened in our parish.

I'm convinced that many married couples break up in divorce because they never did enough healthy breaking up as teens. They never gained the freedom, confidence, and knowledge about love and about themselves that they needed for a permanent married relationship. These attributes are achieved by having lived out a variety of previous relationships.

The more universal, scriptural message in this approach to breaking up is to trust the endings of things as much as the beginnings. Look again at the above passage from John. Young people who cling to relationships in defiance of their own growth feel a terrible aloneness. If they can be encouraged, when the time comes, to trust the letting go, they will find an expanding capacity to live and to love rising within them.

An Open Letter to Magic Johnson

"You are the light of the world. Put your light on a lamp-stand where it will shine for everyone." (See Matthew 5:14–15.)

Dear Magic Johnson,

I enjoyed your appearance on the "Arsenio Hall Show" last Friday night. You were in top form, and I think you connected well with America's young people.

I was impressed by your generous intentions and your courage. But I have to say it—I think you're making a tragic mistake. I would join you in handing my sons and daughter a condom if I thought it could save their lives. But I have come to believe that the false reassurance provided by condoms is more likely to kill them than protect them.

In our state some towns have started down this tragic road with you. Great intentions, but devastating results. Why devastating? When a high school administration or a big star says, "Use condoms to have safe sex," young people will listen. But in reality, the message they get promotes sex as much as it promotes safety. The decision about having sex is on their minds a lot more than the decision about using condoms, and your appealing voice quite obviously exerts an influence on both decisions. Is it possible that you're putting more, not less, of our young people at risk for AIDS by urging them to use condoms?

I work with teenagers, and part of my job is to follow research on adolescent behavior. Here are three findings from research on the behavior of teenagers who have received birth-control counseling from school-based family-planning clinics:

- Teens who received birth-control counseling were one and one-half times more likely to start having intercourse at age fourteen than were teens who had not received counseling.

- Among sexually active females who received contraceptives, sexual activity increased one and one-half times.
- There was a net increase of 50 to 120 pregnancies per 1000 teenage clients.

And here is a startling statistic about condom effectiveness among adolescents: The standard condom failure rate of 10 to 20 percent becomes 20 to 40 percent for teens. (All of the statistics stated come from *AIDS and Adolescents*, by Linda Thayer [Boston: Saint Paul Books and Media, 1992], pages 15, 19, 21.)

Apparently the main effect of birth-control counseling is that it helps teens feel safer about having sex. That sense of false security is actually causing the rate of sexual activity and of "unsafe" sexual activity to go up. We know that when the teen pregnancy rate goes up, the rate of exposure to HIV, the virus that causes AIDS, also goes up.

Let's also remember that these pregnancy statistics only tell us about unsafe sex during a young woman's fertile time of the month, and HIV infection can happen any day of the month. Here is the bottom line of all these statistics: *Many young people may get infected with HIV tonight because of the influence of condoms on their sexual activity.*

Few adult voices are getting through to teens about the risks of sexual activity. Young people struggle with an enormous decision and face enormous danger. You could warn a lot of them about that danger and show them safe ground. You could urge them not to have premarital sex. They would accept that from you. Then you would be truly saving lives.

Resource 1–F: Permission to reproduce this resource is granted.

What Sex Does for and Against Love

"Has no one condemned you? . . . Neither do I condemn you. Go, [and] from now on do not sin any more." (John 8:10–11, NAB)

Dear young seekers of happiness in love,

I came of age in the 1960s, when free love was a fervently held value among the young. I write as one whose search for happiness included sex outside of marriage. I did my learning, like many others of my generation, the hard way—by experiencing the consequences of that value.

You will notice that I offer these personal conclusions with a certain urgency. I write as one who loves you and wants you to find a better road—a road to happiness.

You will also notice that the things I say agree quite well with the urgent message about sex and love that the church expresses to young people. The church's response to the free-love attitude is the same as Jesus' response to the woman who was accused of having sex outside of marriage—not condemnation, but guidance to stop self-destructive behavior.

That message from the church did eventually help me, and I want to pass on that help to you. However, let me make one thing clear. Despite my eagerness, as your older brother in the church, to convey certain values and realities to you, please know that your right and duty to see and decide for yourself about what you hear is also sacred. Please receive these observations in that spirit.

Here is the first conclusion that I have reached: *Sex within marriage does a lot for love and brings about four great blessings that the church has always emphasized:*

1. **Intimate lovemaking:** Sexual intercourse releases feelings of boundless love that can blossom within marriage, but that can only be frustrated and suppressed outside of marriage—by the severe limitation of lovers whose commitment is limited. Within marriage, sex nudges the heart open. Outside of marriage, sex gradually closes the heart. When that pattern of sexual dull-heartedness gets established in young adulthood, it is hard to break, and true closeness can remain elusive.

2. **Conception of new life:** Babies born within marriage usually have the great emotional advantage of having both a mother and a father to grow up with. For that reason, both the Hebrew Scriptures and the Christian Testament have always treated sex outside of marriage as harmful and therefore sinful. When marriage surrounds sex, conception and birth are more likely to be occasions of joy for both parents and children.

3. **Mutual respect:** The pope has cautioned against lust in marriage, and he has taken a lot of flak and even ridicule for it. But he's right. When sex takes over and dominates lovemaking, whether inside or outside marriage, true and deep intimacy cannot occur. Couples who do not control sex during courtship often cannot control it in their marriage. For them, marriage remains a disappointment. Sex can only contribute to love when love, and not sex, is allowed to rule the relationship.

Courtship is the time to prepare a foundation of love and shared spirituality that is sturdy enough to handle all the ups and downs of life—including sex. When sex comes before marriage, that foundation remains incomplete.

4. Awesome reality: In the United States, we often learn our attitudes about sex from movies and television. And what we typically see is a celebration of unmarried sex with low-level commitment. Getting pregnant usually does not enter the picture. This means that emotionally we have been trained for an unreal kind of sex that ignores the "facts of life." In marriage we have a chance to break out of that illusion and get in touch with the awesome reality of sex. When pregnancy is no longer an unthinkable disaster, we can recover an inner wholeness and a sense that the power of mutual attraction is part of the miraculous power of conceiving a new person.

Here is the second conclusion that I have reached: *Sex without marriage works consistently against love.*

Especially since the dawn of effective birth control, society's message has been that unmarried sex between consenting adults does no harm, and that love can now be free of any fear. But the church's message to the world is that unmarried sex is wrong precisely because practical experience has shown that it does do great harm—to our country, to couples, and to the individual.

Harm to our country: Unmarried sex has led to four epidemics:
* *Unwed mothers with fatherless children and unwed fathers with motherless children:* This situation is tough on both parents and children. According to U.S. Census Bureau estimates for 1991, seventeen million of the sixty-five million children under age eighteen in the United States

are raised by a single parent (quoted in *Youthworker Update* [January 1993]: 4).
* *AIDS:* AIDS is the sixth leading cause of death among fifteen- to twenty-four-year-olds, and between 1990 and 1992, AIDS cases among adolescents increased by 77 percent (Donna Futterman and Karen Hein, "Medical Care of HIV-Infected Adolescents," *AIDS Clinical Care* [December 1992]: 1).
* *Abortion:* There are about four thousand abortions per day in the United States; abortion has now become simply a back-up form of birth control ("Roe v. Wade is Finished," *New Covenant* [July–August 1992]: 9).
* *Divorce:* Half of all marriages break up, and the greatest cause is unfaithfulness, that is, people who act on the value that love feelings alone are a sufficient basis for sex (Diane Colasanto and James Shriver, "Middle-Aged Face Marital Crisis," *Gallup Poll News Service* [1 May 1989]: 1).

The direct cause of all four epidemics is people of all ages who tell one another there is no harm in having sex as long as you feel love.

Harm to couples: Sex has an undermining effect on unmarried relationships because of the following:
* Sex in unmarried relationships tends to destroy the relationships because of the stress it creates between the partners.
* Sex brings out an instinctive need to bond with a trust that will not be broken—a trust that is usually absent in unmarried relationships.
* Unmarried sexual relationships constantly call up expectations communicated by sex that are then frustrated because there is no commitment to count on.
* The need to try to meet the expectations activated by sex deprives developing unmarried relationships of the chance to

build a foundation of friendship. That friendship can grow only with freedom from the emotional demands and expectations of sex.

Harm to the individual: Unmarried sex stunts growth because of these reasons:

- It cuts off the freedom, searching, and learning that are essential to a complete preparation for adulthood.
- Broken relationships that were sexually active can be the emotional equivalent of divorce and leave great scarring.
- People often have sex out of loneliness and express in sexual activity what is actually a need to open up and be known as a person. The complications of sex then crowd out the heart's true need, which gets lost.
- Knowing that unmarried sex is against the teachings of Jesus usually turns Christian young people who choose to be sexually active away from Jesus. They often stop listening to him in other areas of their life as well.

Those are conclusions I have come to, thanks to the gentle guidance of the church, over my painful years of searching. I offer my views as a gift, and the gift I ask in return is your honest and searching response to them.

2

A "Battle of the Sexes": Forming Young Hearts for Sturdy Relationships

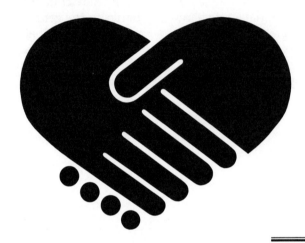

Adult North Americans in the 1990s are having a hard time keeping their love lives together. Confusion about sex and love is rampant, and the effects of this confusion on young people are enormous. When the love problems of parents rob children of a stable home life, that same damaging confusion gets passed on. It shapes the developing sexual values of the next generation, and the cycle continues.

Young people need instruction about love, but that catechesis is not easy to deliver. Along with confused values about love, young people bring another inheritance from the culture—a veneer of false sophistication. They, along with many adult Americans, believe that they are quite enlightened and liberated regarding sexuality—a foolish conceit. Even a brief look at what is happening to us ought to have everyone urgently questioning our commonly held ideas about love. But little such questioning is taking place in our adult culture, and it's certainly not happening among teens. So what catechetical approach do we take?

Let's set aside catechetical *content* for a moment. I have, first, a catechetical *style* to propose—a kind of approach that I call prophetic. The tone is boldness. The purpose is to pierce the know-it-all cultural veneer with undeniable facts and figures that reveal how shallow our culture actually is about love and sex.

Young people need to be warned—just as the prophets of old warned people—that if they continue to live the values our culture teaches them, their capacity to express their genuine sexuality and to draw close in love to others will be greatly impaired. In fact, to mature in wholeness, they need to become sharp critics of prevailing love attitudes in the United States.

However, young people may think that their church cannot teach them anything about love, especially romantic love. Yet, the wisdom of the church leads the way to relationships that are very close, beautiful, and happy.

These are bold statements, but we have a bold Gospel. And before young people will open up to its healing help, they need to sense our confidence in its wisdom. The point is that the wisdom of Christ and his church can reclaim for a love relationship between a man and a woman a sacredness and a beauty that is in fact sacramental. Coaching young people with that catechetical wisdom can enable them to practice, in their short-term relationships, a way of loving that can bring them free, responsible, and even skilled to the sacramental and permanent bond of marriage.

Catechesis on Sexuality and Relationships

The following is a two-part catechetical program consisting of two training sessions on relations between the sexes. The program presents the Catholic church's values (on sex) as prophetic, healing remedies that will enable young people to become whole adults, uncorrupted by the sex values of our culture.

Part A

"Battle of the Sexes"

Introduction

I introduce the session with the following explanation:

Tonight's activity is called the "Battle of the Sexes," but before we wage the actual battle, I want to explain its purpose. We will be exploring the subject of sexuality. Does that mean the subject is sex? Yes, that's part of it, but sexuality includes more than sexual activity—a lot more! The word *sexuality* means "the style of maleness or femaleness with which you relate to people, especially members of the other sex."

The purpose of the "Battle of the Sexes" is to help you further develop your sexuality. The definition of well-developed sexuality is "the ability to relate to people, especially those of the other sex, in a way that makes both parties happy." Does that seem to be a fairly simple and attainable goal? Well, I have a statement to make about sexuality in the United States.

Many American men and women today have poorly developed sexualities. The statistics speak for themselves: About 50 percent of American adults cannot keep their marriages together [Colasanto and Shriver, "Middle-Aged Face Marital Crisis," p. 1]. They don't know how to relate so as to enhance each other's happiness. And a lot of other marriages that don't actually break up are very unhappy.

What has happened? Where has this crisis come from? Why haven't American men and women come into adulthood with a mature and balanced ability to relate to the other sex? What has caused their sexualities to become so poorly developed or so badly damaged?

I'm going to leave you in suspense of the answers to those fairly crucial questions. You will probably find some clues yourself as you go through this "Battle of the Sexes."

Our purpose for staging the battle and its following discussion is fourfold. We want to help all of you gain the following:
- a better sense of your own emerging sexuality
- a clear idea of how you can develop your own personal style of masculinity or femininity so that you can successfully relate to others, especially those of the other sex
- an awareness of specific ways to make relationships between the sexes more successful—that is, more interesting, challenging, growth-producing, and caring
- an understanding of how early sexual activity impacts your developing sexuality

Here's one final point for any of you who may be considering a religious vocation: Don't back off and say, "Oh well, if I am going to be celibate, this session isn't for me." On the contrary, this session is especially for you.

Attractive maleness or femaleness is especially important for priests, brothers, and sisters if they are going to be successful in their call to love everyone. Okay, any questions about what you've heard so far?

Step 1 | **Separation**

For step 1, I direct the young people as follows:

Let the "Battle of the Sexes" begin. Young women, young men, please go to opposite sides of the room. [When they have separated, I continue.] Your sexuality involves knowing what is unique about being male or female, knowing what qualities you have going for you, and gaining confidence in your masculinity or femininity. So pair off with someone of the same sex and discuss this question: *What do you like best about the company of other members of your own sex?* Record on a sheet of paper the likable qualities you come up with.

[After they have done this, I go on.] Now join with another pair of people of your own sex and share your lists with one another.

Step 2 | **Struggles**

Here are the directions I give for step 2:

The sexes are different in wonderful, challenging ways. Often we drive one another crazy. Our traits and tendencies do not always match well, at least not without some effort. So here is a question for you foursomes, and be honest: *In your relationships with the other sex, what do you find frustrating, perplexing, or difficult about them?* Make a list. Be candid but respectful.

[When they are done with their lists, I continue.] Now, men and women, gather as separate large groups and make a composite list of what you find difficult about the other sex. Then pick a spokesperson who you feel will present your list with flair. [I give them several minutes and then call for their lists.]

Women's spokesperson, your list please. [She reads it—no discussion is allowed—but it may be impossible to stop some laughter.]

Men's spokesperson, your list please. [He reads it. Again, there may be some laughter.]

[After the lists have been read, spend some time identifying any false or unfair generalizations about either sex.]

Now form two long lines, the women facing the men. When I say "Go," walk toward one another and find a partner of the other sex. Then stand right there and ask each other this question: *From your experience, what do you have a hard time understanding about the way members of the other sex think?* [They form their lines, and then I say "Go."]

[When they have finished discussing the question, I proceed.] Now find a new partner of the other sex nearby and discuss this question: *In your experience of the traits or tendencies of members of the other sex, which of these traits do you find the hardest to relate to?* [I let them discuss the question before moving on to step 3.]

Step 3 | **Affirmations**

The directions I give for step 3 are these:

Now go back to your same-sex foursomes. [I continue after they have done this.] The sexes are also different in some wonderfully appealing ways—in ways that go beyond the obvious physical attractions. Please discuss this question and then list your group's responses on a sheet of paper: *From your experience, what are the qualities you like best, the special strengths you see, in the other sex?*

[After they have compiled their lists, I continue.] Once again, bring your lists to your large same-sex group and pool them into a single composite list. Pick a new spokesperson to announce your findings. [They do so, and then I go on.]

Both sides, please step forward and prepare to listen to the reading of the lists. [They do so.]

Women's spokesperson, your list please. [She reads it.]
Men's spokesperson, your list please. [He reads it.]

Now form two lines facing one another, and at my signal, approach one another and find a partner of the other sex. Then take turns completing this sentence: *From my experience, what I like best about the other sex is . . .* [They form their lines, and then I say "Go."]

[After a few minutes, I continue.] Next, find a new other-sex partner and complete this statement: *From my experience, the special strengths I see in the other sex are . . .* [They do so.]

Step 4 | **Families**

For step 4, I give the young people the following directions:

> Now please gather as same-sex foursomes again. Then join with one other-sex foursome to form mixed families of eight. [They do so.]
>
> The four women in each group will now go and get cider and cups for eight, and the four men in each group will now go and get chips and dip for eight. After retrieving the snacks, gather your family around a table, eat and drink together, and share your reactions to your encounters with the other sex. [I let them talk and snack for a while before continuing.]
>
> Next, pick a moderator. The moderator will now go and get a "moderator sheet" listing the following four questions, which you are to discuss as a family—as brothers and sisters. [You will need to prepare and photocopy a moderator sheet listing these questions.]
>
> *a.* Given the differences we have named, what does it take for women and men to be good friends with strong feelings for one another—feelings that are not necessarily romantic?
> *b.* What do you think men and women have to learn from one another in friendship?
>
> [After the first two questions, we sometimes take a break. Then the families discuss the other two questions.]
>
> *c.* Two commonly practiced values in romantic relationships are (1) "I have to make whatever sacrifices it takes to keep the relationship going," and (2) "I have to do whatever it takes to ensure that we both keep growing into full persons." How do people put each of those values into practice? How important is each value in comparison to the other?
> *d.* When something upsetting happens in a love relationship, what are some typical negative ways of responding? What do you think are some positive ways of responding?

Step 5 | **Clues**

Everyone comes back together as one large group, and I ask them:

> Please think back over your encounters with others during this session and list any clues you've found about what is

missing in the styles of relating between the sexes in the United States.

I then list on a sheet of newsprint the group's insights about the troubles plaguing the love lives of most Americans.

The first session takes just an hour and a half. Step 5 sums up the session and provides a link with part B.

Part B | ## The Meaning of the "Battle of the Sexes"

Steps 6 through 8 explain the model of sexuality development underlying the "Battle of the Sexes." My style of presentation is one of catechetical authority; please recall the boldness I proposed at the beginning of this chapter. However, you may be wondering what sources I have for my content—my "facts of life." I used these sources:

- The church's ancient and unwavering insistence that sex without marriage does great harm.
- Bitter lessons from my personal experience of coming of age in a generation that threw off sexual restraint in favor of free love.
- Much counseling and reflection on the effects of sexual activity and sexual self-control on the quality of adolescent maturation.
- Simple observation of the devastation in our society that has resulted from people's living of a "liberated" adult sexuality.

Step 6 | ### Witness

I introduce the witness step this way:

> People must go through four distinct phases to develop a full sexuality, that is, a healthy responsiveness to the other sex. In the United States, these stages are often being skipped, and the result is a generation of adults who find themselves unprepared and incompetent when they get to the marriage relationship. You have already identified some of what is missing. In a moment, we will spell out all four developmental phases, along with what is hampering people from going through all of them. But first, let's hear from someone who knows from personal experience what is damaging us as Americans in our sexuality. Sexuality, you may recall, means "our ability to relate to others, especially the other sex, in a way that makes both parties happy."

At this point, I introduce an adult who came of age practicing sex-without-marriage values. This person reports the results of the "free-love" lifestyle from his or her own experience.

Witness stories have terrific impact not only because of their powerful illustrations of the self-damaging effects of premarital sex but also because of the evident love of people willing to tell their story discreetly but candidly so as to warn the next generation to take a different road.

If no adult is available to offer such a witness, proceed to the next step.

Step 7

Talk

The talk I give for step 7 is as follows:

The key to the riddle of our country's difficulty with marriage is the fact that most Americans now become sexually active before they are psychologically or emotionally ready. Sexual activity interrupts the development of sexuality. Here's how that interruption works:

When you become sexually active, you become functionally and sexually an adult. Adolescence is a period of growth and major change in who you are—and that includes who you are with the other sex. During adolescence you find your sexuality—not quickly, but gradually, through a lot of relating and reflecting, constantly trying out new and better ways to be male or female. This experimentation takes you naturally through four distinct stages on your way to a masculine or a feminine sexuality that is well developed and provides a sound basis for healthy love relationships. However, you can miss those four growth stages by stepping across into sexually active adulthood, taking with you only as much of your developing sexuality as you have going for you at that time. That premature entry into sexual adulthood is the reason so many American men and women come of age with an immature sexuality and fare so poorly in the real world of marriage.

In a few moments, we will talk more about how interruption of the maturation process affects young people's sexuality. But first, let's look at the four stages of development of a healthy sexuality. These stages are *same-sex friendship, other-sex friendship, romantic intimacy,* and *spiritual intimacy.*

The titles of the four stages are each written on a sheet of paper. I tape each sheet to the wall after reading aloud its definition from column 1 of resource 2–A, "Sexuality," or explaining its definition in my own words. After the stages are defined and discussed, I make the following points:

1. Young people go through all four stages of development gradually during adolescence. This development is part of the natural momentum for physical and psychological growth that continues from childhood, and it needs plenty of time to reach maturity before it ends when we step into adult functioning and establish our adult personalities.
2. When we choose to become sexually active, our sexual desires and pursuits depend on and make full use of the relational capacities we have developed thus far. At that point, we cause a clicking into place of our sexuality at whatever developmental stage we have reached.
3. Once launched into sexual activity, few young adults will be able or willing to stop and backtrack so as to make room for further development of their sexuality. Backtracking is extremely difficult because it calls not only for abstinence but also for breaking down and rebuilding relational habits.
4. The sex act triggers the psychological need for permanent commitment, and our reproductive system uses that bonding impulse to prepare a place for children. In couples who are sexually active prematurely, that deep biological and psychological response to having sex usually causes one partner to grasp for total commitment and the other to run from it. These opposite reactions put tremendous strain on relationships, and they help shape the way the partners involved will subsequently relate to members of the other sex.

Resource 2–A, "Sexuality" matches each developmental stage (column 1) with a corresponding underdeveloped adult sexuality (column 2) that may surface as a result of premature sexual activity. I introduce the underdeveloped sexualities as follows:

A high percentage of adult Americans are frozen into one of four distinct underdeveloped forms of sexuality, depending on how far they had developed when they decided to become sexually active. The four underdeveloped adult sexualities are actually counterfeits of the healthy capacities the young adults were ready to learn and needed to learn before they stepped into adulthood.

The titles of the four underdeveloped adult sexualities are each written on a sheet of paper. I tape each sheet to the wall next to its corresponding stage of development after reading its description from column 2 of resource 2–A.

Step 8 | **Discussion**

When all four stages of sexual development and the four counterfeits that negate them have been named, displayed, and explained, I invite the group to offer comments, ask questions, or raise objections. The following points usually arise, but I address them even if they do not:

- Premarital sex leads to a lot of thoughtless marriage decisions. Here's why: Once sexual involvement has begun, couples lose the clarity needed to make that all-important decision about who to marry because their most immediate feelings tell them that the choice has already been made and that it will hurt too much to step back and discuss the pros and cons of staying together.
- Some people in youth ministry have begun referring to a "second virginity" for young people who step back from sexual activity, celebrate the sacrament of reconciliation, and get back to being an adolescent.
- The reason so few engaged couples postpone sexual involvement and take the time needed for completing their sexual development with a strong spiritual foundation is that American culture is presently so anti-spiritual. Many couples have no awareness that God and faith are crucial to their future marital happiness and therefore to their preparation for marriage.
- Apart from a community that supports the Christian vision of healthy sexual development, it is next to impossible to resist the huge pressure to have sex before marriage and thus complete all four growth stages.
- Spiritual intimacy is a desirable and appropriate kind of love relationship for men and women who are attracted to each other but for whom marriage would be inappropriate. This type of love fosters much growth in both partners. Saint Francis and Saint Clare had this kind of relationship.
- Spiritual intimacy in premarital relationships helps avoid unwise marriage decisions. Partners owe it to themselves and to each other to thoroughly examine whether they

have common values and shared goals that are mutually inspiring enough to support each other in them for life. Partner choices without such total dialog are built on fantasy and luck—bad luck as often as not.

To close the discussion and the evening, I ask people what they have gained from the "Battle of the Sexes" and the follow-up presentation. Then I hand out copies of resource 2–A for the young people to take home with them.

After one "Battle of the Sexes," I recall being approached in the hallway by several young people who discreetly told me that the counterfeits described just where they were stuck. They urgently wanted to know about second virginity. I explained that the sacrament of reconciliation has all the elements they need: confession, a commitment to chastity, and the words of Jesus, such as those to the frightened young woman who was taken in adultery but rescued by his intervention: "'Has no one condemned you? . . . Neither do I condemn you. Go, [and] from now on do not sin any more'" (John 8:10–11, NAB).

Resource 2–A

Sexuality

Column 1
Four stages of adolescent development that
build a mature sexuality:

Column 2
Four underdeveloped adult forms of sexuality that result from premature sexual
activity:

1. Same-Sex Friendship ◄──►
When good friends of your own sex like
you for who you are, then you can be
yourself. You no longer have to try to
prove anything to them. Same-sex friendships can give you the confidence you
need to break out of popular stereotypes of
masculinity and femininity. The strong
bond of friendship also frees you to express yourself the way you want to, and
even to experiment and coach one another. In other words, friendship allows you to
develop your own comfortable style of
being yourself as a male or female. This
unique sense of your own relaxed masculinity or femininity lets your attractiveness emerge. You will be aware of this
attractiveness and later bring it to your
other-sex friendships.

Exploitive Sexuality
Sexual activity has little to do with the
actual partner, because the real need and
purpose is to prove the power of one's sexuality to same-sex friends and to oneself.
Such unkindness and misuse of another
person dehumanizes the heart, and the
capacity for friendship between the sexes is
reduced.

Here are some supporting statistics: According to a talk given by Dr. Peter Benson
at the Hartford Conference of the New
England Consultants for Youth Ministry,
50 percent of teen pregnancies are reported
to have been conceived when one or both
of the partners were drunk.

The FBI reports that 33 percent of American women will be sexually assaulted in
their lifetime (Tom Keogh, "A Well-Placed
Kick," *New Age Journal* [August 1992]: 60).

2. Other-Sex Friendship ◄──►
When other-sex friendships develop and
males and females learn to open up and
confide in one another, that heart-to-heart
communication offers a great opportunity
to learn from one another. Other-sex
friendships also help people develop the
ability to overcome a certain distance or
discomfort with the other sex, which
many people carry with them all of their
adult life. Though building a bond of
friendship between the sexes may be challenging, the rewards can be great. A lasting
appreciation and mutual respect that goes
beyond your particular friend develops. In
other words, you discover what there is to
love in the other sex. The attitudes and

Casual Sexuality
Sexual activity is a form of social recreation
that avoids personal closeness as being
vulnerable and weak. Behind a mask of
sophistication, perhaps because of prior
hurt, lies loneliness and an inability to
bring deep feeling, intimacy, or commitment—or love—to other-sex relationships.

The following are some alarming statistics: Nearly 40 percent of today's twenty-
year-old American females were pregnant
as teenagers—the highest rate of any in-
dustrialized country in the world (John S.
Nelson et al., *Readings in Youth Ministry*,
vol. 1, *Foundations* [Washington, DC: National Federation for Catholic Youth Ministry, 1986], p. 66).

relational skills you gain from the relation-ship open and strengthen your heart. These skills are a tremendous asset when the time comes for romantic love.

3. Romantic Intimacy ◄——►
When you fall in love, your whole out-look—and sometimes your whole life—changes. The beautiful qualities of your partner, which grip you so deeply, can unlock new possibilities in your own per-sonality. When love is true, the intense need for each other can awaken the courage to be totally honest with each other, instead of hiding behind masks and playing games of deception. If you love each other enough to really seek out, find, and be as close to each other as you are to yourself, then a blossoming of your real selves begins to occur. That wonderful sense of growth and mutual discovery, as long as its lasts, is the purpose of intimacy. And when that growth and mutual discov-ery ends, you come away more fully your-self.

4. Spiritual Intimacy ◄——►
Couples can share in each other's spiritual growth. The relationship each of you has with God then challenges and enriches your partner. The feeling of mutual love is not allowed to become exclusive, and new ways to let God's love, guidance, healing, and wisdom into the relationship are dis-covered. The question of marriage then becomes not just a matter of attraction but rather of asking, Does God want the unique lives and paths to which each of us is called to be combined for life? Some great loves are not meant to be great mar-riages. Your love for each other will prompt not a mutual grasping for security, but instead, much prayer and discussion as to whether marriage is best for both parties and whether it is meant to be.

There are about four thousand abortions per day in the United States; abortion has now become simply a backup form of birth control ("Roe v. Wade is Finished," *New Covenant* [July–August 1992]: 9).

Free-Love Sexuality
Sexual involvement expresses strong feel-ings but no commitment. Love chooses and experiences the intense demands of physical closeness instead of the relaxed development of personal closeness. Breakups are devastating, and afterward, the heart will not easily trust again.

Here are some disturbing statistics: About 41 percent of depressed or suicidal college students cite love problems as the cause of their behavior (John S. Westefeld and Susan R. Furr, "Suicide and Depression Among College Students," *Professional Psy-chology: Research and Practice* 18, no. 2 [1987]: 121).

According to Dean Borgman of the Cen-ter for Youth Studies in Wenham, Mas-sachusetts, the average adolescent falls in love three times before marriage.

Unstable Sexuality
The premature grasp for sexual happiness leads to thoughtless marriage decisions. It becomes too difficult to step back and ask these questions: Do our spiritual goals, values, and selves really match up? Is this relationship meant to be? Marriages with no spiritual foundation crack easily.

The following statistics illustrate this trend: Approximately 50 percent of mar-ried women in the United States eventual-ly commit adultery. The figure for men is nearly 67 percent (Joyce Brothers, "Why Wives Have Affairs," *Parade* [18 February 1990]: 4).

3

Civilized Dating:
Care-fullness in Dating Relationships

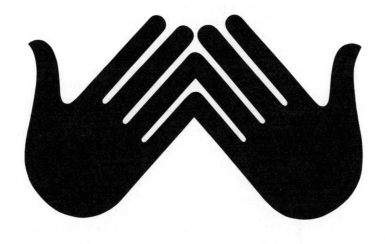

The Problem

At one of our weekly peer leadership meetings, I offered this observation: Teens often get badly hurt in dating relationships, not from any bad intention, but from ignorance about how to treat people right when romantic feelings are involved. That remark met with an outpouring of unanimous and vigorous agreement. One young person summed up the feeling: "You take a risk when you love. You make yourself vulnerable. And if someone is rotten to you, it could be a long time before you trust again."

After much discussion we came to the following conclusions about this problem: dating takes courage, getting close and developing a relationship takes courage, and breaking up also takes courage. That courage deserves to be treated with respect and care, but often in the midst of all the stresses, challenges, and complexities of love relationships, people are not treated very well or very fairly. We agreed that needless harm could be avoided if we could come up with some caring and honest ways to handle the challenges and changes inherent in dating relationships. We were not trying to eliminate all the pain of love—some pain is a healthy and necessary part of growing up and should not be avoided. Rather, we were going after the unnecessary pain that comes from people being inconsiderate and unkind to one another.

The leadership group made a list of specific problem areas—"dating dilemmas"—in which people get mistreated and hurt. That list of situations was then brought to the weekly youth meeting. We asked everyone to go over the list, adding and subtracting items until we had a consensus on what our particular youth group considered to be the toughest dating dilemmas.

An entire Sunday night meeting was needed just to name and list all the different kinds of struggles people were facing. Then it took two more meetings to work on solutions to those dilemmas.

I told the group that their list of dating dilemmas and solutions would be presented in this book, not as *the* list, but rather as an expression of what one youth group had found challenging in the dating process. And I can assure you that anticipating the publication of their list added plenty of extra energy and interest to those discussions. Our purpose was to stimulate other youth groups to make their own lists and to set in motion their own processes of talking, searching, and praying about dating dilemmas.

The process we used to develop our list of dilemmas and solutions, as described above, is quite simple. You may wish to copy it or use a process of your own design.

The following is a summary of our dilemmas and solutions. Again, our solutions are not to be taken as conclusive answers to all dating dilemmas, but they can serve as points of comparison with the dilemmas and solutions your group may wish to develop.

Dating Dilemmas and Solutions

Our list of dilemmas and solutions breaks down into four distinct categories that are common aspects of dating relationships: getting started, going deeper, other people, and breaking up.

The "Getting Started" Aspect

Some Troublesome Attitudes

Dilemma 1: Someone asks you out on the basis of physical attraction; she or he expresses no interest in building a friendship.

Solution: Sometimes the best response is a firm "no thank you," but it depends on the person. Sometimes underneath the prompting of physical attraction, a caring heart is awkwardly expressing itself. Even when physical attraction seems to be the primary motive, accepting one date and proposing the building of a friendship might be worth a try. However, when dating doesn't reach for friendship, it quickly breaks down. Friendship is the solid foundation for good dating relationships.

Dilemma 2: You want to have a girlfriend or a boyfriend as a convenience, like a car or a VCR, just because it's harder socially to be alone.

Solution: Treating a person like a possession is emotionally abusive. Fight it in yourself. Fight it in your partner. If convenience is the primary basis for a dating relationship, get out of it, or you will both get hurt.

Dilemma 3: You are asked out by someone you're not interested in romantically, and you don't know how to be honest and refuse the date without rejecting the person.

Solution: Dating is a trial-and-error method of discovering the qualities (chemistry) that attract you to another person. But it's hard to discern qualities in another person from surface impressions. If you feel the person asking you out is a good human being, you can accept the date on a friendly basis, to find out whether the relationship feels right. If there's no special electricity, you should not accept a second date. And do not give any vague excuses; that's lying. Explain why you don't want to continue dating the person. For example, "I don't feel that continued dating is going to work out." That way you don't build false hopes. The truth spoken with real care is freeing for everyone.

Dilemma 4: You are really down on yourself because you don't have a boyfriend or a girlfriend. You begin to feel that something must be wrong with you.

Solution: Equating your self-worth with your love life is a big mistake. There is a lot more to you and a lot more to life than being someone's partner. Let love come when and however it wishes, and remember that there is a lot of time ahead for that to happen. Your main concern right now is to keep on finding and bringing out more and more of the treasures you have within you. And you can do that in all kinds of relationships, not just dating relationships. Do not fall into the trap of worshiping love. Put your trust in Jesus and in yourself. (See "Love-Coaching Resource for Session 1: The Two Faces of Love" on page 17.)

The "Going Deeper" Aspect

Some Troublesome Behaviors

Dilemma 1: The person you're dating starts behaving in a way you feel is wrong, but you don't want to offend her or him by saying something about it.

Solution: If your partner behaves in a way you feel is wrong, you'll be supporting the behavior if you don't speak up. True, it's a risk to bring the matter up. No matter how gently you express your feelings, you might scare the person away. But on the other hand, you just might open up a whole new trust because you cared enough and dared to speak. Speak up and do not worry about what might happen. Even if the behavior turns out to be harmless, a relationship that stifles honesty is worthless.

Dilemma 2: The person you're dating won't open up, won't let you in on his or her real feelings, won't get close, and won't allow any communication to go beyond surface things.

Solution: People often complain that their partner won't open up his or her inner feelings and thoughts. But sometimes people are so busy expressing their own feelings and thoughts that they don't really invite other people to share; they don't really offer a listening heart. A good way to initiate some sharing would be to ask, "How important is it to you that we learn to get beyond surface communication?"

Dilemma 3: When something difficult happens between you and your partner, one of you turns off—or blows up—and in either case, refuses to talk about it and work things out.

Solution: Handling hurt when it comes from someone you care for is love's greatest challenge. People normally clam up or explode. Pray first, to regain a positive attitude, then quietly state your feelings. After you have stated your feelings, ask a lot of questions and listen carefully to the other person. When both partners are believers, a time of hurt feelings is a good time to join hands and pray together.

Dilemma 4: The person you're dating doesn't respect your limits on how far to go sexually and just keeps pushing.

Solution: Every dating couple has to mutually agree to their limits regarding sexual activity, or the relationship will go sour. Disagreements must be worked out and agreements made, or an important part of dating will become a battleground that will erode otherwise-good feelings for each other. In making an agreement about the limits of sexual activity, both partners should be aware that "going all the way" in a dating relationship will undermine rather than enhance the growth of friendship, and it will make breaking up a great deal more painful, even personally destructive. (See "Love-Coaching Resource for Session 5: Breaking Up" on page 21.)

The "Other People" Aspect

Some Troublesome Questions

Dilemma 1: How much should I tell a friend about what's happening between me and my girlfriend or boyfriend?
Solution: If your friend is trustworthy, you should feel free to tell him or her anything you want or need to. Confiding in a friend may be a necessary way to sort out your feelings about what is happening in the relationship and about how to proceed. Let your partner in on any conversations with other friends that involve him or her so that trust will be maintained and both of you can benefit from the conversations.

Dilemma 2: What if my girlfriend or boyfriend gets possessive and becomes jealous of time spent with other friends or in activities that do not include her or him?
Solution: Possessiveness is selfish and destructive and should not be tolerated. Nip it in the bud, and if it continues to grow, end the relationship. A possessive or jealous person will deprive you of other relationships you need for growth. Possessiveness and jealousy are signs that love is lacking. A healthy love relationship has room for lots of other friendships.

Dilemma 3: How much should I let myself be influenced by what my friends think about my boyfriend or girlfriend?
Solution: Listen carefully to whatever your friends want to tell you. Then take it all to prayer, knowing that they may be way off base or right on target. Ask Christ to show you which is the case, and only then draw your own conclusions.

Dilemma 4: What if my parents don't like my girlfriend or boyfriend?
Solution: Listen with an open mind to what your parents have to say. Some parents, whether from their own successes or their own failures in love, will have a lot of wisdom to offer you about your dating decisions. On the other hand, some parents might not be all that helpful if they cannot get beyond their own experience and see yours for what it is. In either case, ask your parents to stand beside you and coach you

instead of trying to make your decisions for you. In some cases, your parents may see a danger that you don't and order you to break off the relationship. If this happens, you need to obey them because at high-school age, you're still under their authority. If you deeply feel they're wrong, go to God and put the matter in God's hands. Ask for the light to see the situation through God's eyes and the courage to do what is best for all involved.

The "Breaking Up" Aspect

Some Troublesome Reactions

Dilemma 1: You've lost "that lovin' feeling," but you keep the relationship going because you don't want all the pain and hassle of breaking up.

Solution: The turmoil of breaking up is painful but healthy. It frees up both partners to enter new dating relationships that can bring new growth. Most dating relationships have only so much to offer, and it's an act of kindness and courage to say so when you realize it's time to move on. (See "Love-Coaching Resource for Session 5: Breaking Up" on page 21.)

Dilemma 2: You want to end the relationship, so you act cold and hope your partner "gets the picture."

Solution: The great majority of teen love relationships will break up. Breaking up is a normal process, so it's good to learn how. A well-handled breakup is talked out, not just acted out. In fact, a healthy breakup may take several long conversations. The more both partners understand each other, the freer it will leave them. During the breakup both partners need to share what they have gained from being together. If friendship was truly developed during the dating relationship, it will actually be strengthened by going through the pain of breaking up in a considerate and open way. (See "Love-Coaching Resource for Session 5: Breaking Up" on page 21.)

Dilemma 3: You're told "it's over," but you refuse to believe it and won't let go.

Solution: Refusing to let go when that's what the other person really wants is selfish. You will only do harm to yourself and your partner by hanging on. If your attachment feels like a life-or-death loss, pray about the situation and ask Christ to take you beyond it. He will see you through the sadness and help you make new beginnings. (See "Love-Coaching Resource for Session 5: Breaking Up" on page 21.)

Dilemma 4: At the worst possible time and in the worst possible place, you get the bad news that your partner wants out.

Solution: The reason nearly all teen romantic relationships break up is that both partners, at this age, still have a lot to learn about love. So even at the beginning, expect that the dating relationship may well break up. When the time comes, if you feel and know that the relationship is over, choose a time and place free from a lot of other pressures—a time and place where both of you can freely air all the feelings involved and be able to leave the relationship behind with hope, confidence, and a good feeling about each other. (See "Love-Coaching Resource for Session 5: Breaking Up" on page 21.)

Our group worked hard and had a lot of fun developing our list of dating dilemmas and solutions. I am convinced that all the openness and effort they invested did more to build up and encourage sound love values in themselves than any amount of adult teaching on those same values could ever have produced. So I encourage you to put your group to work too. And bring out our list only to see if our groups agree.

I will close with two Gospel verses that seem to shed light on the search for solutions to dating dilemmas. The first passage is, "'Do to others as you would have them do to you'" (Luke 6:31, NAB). In romantic relationships we can be tempted to act selfishly because our needs, our feelings, and our very hope of happiness seem to be on the line. But our actual happiness also depends on caring deeply about the effects our decisions have on others as well as on ourselves. The second passage is, "'The truth will set you free'" (John 8:32, NAB). When strong feelings are involved, like those in a dating relationship, we can be tempted to withhold the truth because the truth sometimes hurts. But if expressed with real caring, the truth opens the way for the communication and the learning that are necessary for personal growth and healthy relationships.

Pastoral Postscript | **A Larger Perspective on Dating**

A majority of teens will welcome the chance to think through their dating dilemmas. But what about teens in your group who don't date? All this attention to love relationships can easily make them feel left out, or worse, that there's something wrong with them—unless you send a different message.

Here's the message I recommend:

Romantic love is one absorbing area for teen growth. But it would be stereotyping to suggest that it is the main concern of all young people. The main concern of some teens is mastering a sport, becoming a musician, or some other area of accomplishment. Some teens make non-romantic friendships their priority. Others focus their energies on building a better world or on sharing their faith.

The American emphasis on teen dating does get a bit obsessive, and it can be a trap. Those whose growth as teens calls them to pursue interests other than dating need to shake off the oppressive idea that there's something wrong with not dating. The truly liberating idea that our young people need to hear is that every young life unfolds uniquely.

4

An Open Heart:
A Workshop on Homosexuality

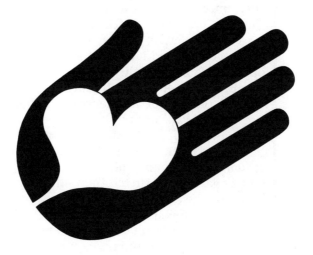

This chapter offers two sessions on homosexuality. Session 1 introduces the issue. It has two specific purposes:

a. to introduce the participants to the various ways that all teens are confronted by homosexuality

b. to help the participants develop a contract of mutual respect, which is necessary for the second session

Session 2 is a workshop that deals with the homosexuality issue in some depth and involves a high degree of group participation. The workshop's success depends on the participants' commitment, forged in session 1, to bring mutual respect to this controversial issue.

Session 1	Introducing the Issue

The introduction that follows is addressed to you as teachers and group leaders, but not only to you. Like the seven resource sheets in chapter 1, this introduction is designed to be heard by the young people. The idea is to let them eavesdrop on an adult perception of an issue as it affects young people and to let the young people's response to that material launch their discussion. Read aloud the introduction as if you are talking to another adult and then distribute copies of it to the participants for their reference in the discussion that follows.

Introduction

Our young people need us to open up the issue of homosexuality. But it's a subject we usually won't touch. The issue is too complex, and we don't feel qualified to comment. Or the issue is too controversial, and we don't feel clear enough on our own feelings about it to be of much help. And besides, we tell ourselves, homosexuality doesn't affect everyone.

But that's not true. Virtually all young people are confronted, one way or another, with homosexuality. They cannot just walk around the issue; so struggle they must—with or without us. Young people need from us the kind of help that the strategies earlier in this book offer on other sexual issues—an invitation to talk openly and think carefully, and a challenge to stretch their minds and gain wisdom for handling the decisions they face.

Yet do all young people really need this discussion? Do all of them have difficult decisions to make about homosexuality? Yes, they all do, and perhaps a case can best be made for running the workshop by explaining four confused responses to homosexuality often detected in many young Catholics.

1. Some young people laugh at homosexual people and regard them not as people at all, but as despicable and subhuman. They may not actually go out of their way to insult or injure someone who they think is gay or lesbian, but their joking disdain is still violent. Under the right conditions, these young people would readily cast their vote or their stone to deprive homosexual people of their civil, and even human, rights. The attitude they've adopted is often mindless and cruel, but it runs deep in our society, and recently it has been given a name—*homophobia*—which means antagonism toward homosexual people.

Unless we as a church find a way, while our young people are still impressionable, to challenge this antagonistic attitude as unchristian and unhealthy, it will take root and become a hate obsession that casts a shadow over their adult life.

2. Other young people are greatly offended by antihomosexual hate and react by taking a strong stand in support of the gay movement, which is gaining strength in our society.

They know that the Catholic church does not approve of homosexual activity, so they unite their voices with the gay movement and label their church as homophobic, thus lumping it in with antihomosexual hate groups.

Young Catholics supporting the gay movement likely don't realize that the church recently defended homosexual civil rights (but not homosexual behavior) by opposing a 1992 referendum to the Oregon state constitution that would have increased discrimination and hostility toward homosexual people. Nor do they know about the church's worldwide efforts on behalf of victims of the AIDS epidemic. These are not the efforts of an antihomosexual church, but our young people don't know about these activities because the news media don't usually report them.

Most young gay-rights supporters haven't read what the church does teach, so they don't know that homosexual people are not being singled out. The church deems many other sexual activities being practiced in our society as unhealthy and harmful, because these practices separate sex from its natural purposes. And many gay-rights supporters also don't know that every word of the church's teaching carries with it great care for the well-being of homosexual people. (That teaching will be explored in session 2.)

In labeling the church as antihomosexual, these young people identify themselves with an anti-Catholic attitude that goes beyond the homosexuality issue. That anti-Catholic attitude is gaining ground in our society. Disdain for "Rome" undermines young people's trust in the rest of church teaching and compromises their personal allegiance to Catholic Tradition.

3. A third group of young people experience occasional homosexual stirrings. They worry about whether those feelings are normal. They don't realize that the vast majority of adolescents do, at times, have homosexual feelings. Instead, their homosexual feelings raise great fears that they are, in fact, homosexual. While that may be true for a small percentage of these teens, the reality is that most of them with homosexual feelings could go either way. Their choices and values are the primary definers of who they are sexually.

Fear of homosexuality also causes teens to suppress natural and healthy feelings of affection for same-sex friends. Learning to express those feelings is an important step of maturation. And fear of homosexuality can freeze that development and cause some young people to pull back from strong and healthy same-sex friendships.

Fear of homosexuality even drives some teens to become heterosexually active just to prove that they aren't gay. And others deny their healthy same-sex love feelings, even from themselves, by parading an exaggerated antihomosexual attitude.

4. Finally, a small percentage of young people are facing more than occasional homosexual feelings. They find themselves exclusively attracted to the same sex, and despite efforts to date other-sex partners, that orientation remains.

These young people are particularly at risk. The U.S. government estimates that one-third of all teenage suicides are related to the difficulties gay and lesbian adolescents face (John F. Tuohey, "The C.D.F. and Homosexuals: Rewriting the Moral Tradition," *America* [12 September 1992]: 138). The prospect of a gay or lesbian adult love life, the fear of rejection by family and friends, the loss of opportunity to have a family, or the mistaken belief that their church condemns them drives many young people to despair.

Gay and lesbian youth are convinced by what they've read or heard that a deep homosexual orientation can never change. They've never heard of Courage and other respected and approved Catholic and Protestant ministries that support homosexual people in happy lives of self-control or in discovering their heterosexuality. And they may not hear of the high success rate of these ministries, because the media consistently refuse to report them, or they dismiss the ministries with the disdainful label of "fundamentalist."

Young people need to know about all these ministries of support. Even more than that, they need to hear and feel from their adult leaders and peers an attitude of loving acceptance as they face this daunting issue.

Society's four main confusions about homosexuality are powerful crosscurrents that tug at our young people. Each one seeks to indoctrinate them with its own persuasive antagonism—against gays and lesbians, against the church, against their own feelings, and against ministries of support and healing.

Our young people need us to open up the subject of homosexuality and create an atmosphere that lets them call into question the unkind, unhealthy, and unthinking views that seek their allegiance. They need to bring their best thinking and their highest ideals to a subject that plays on their fears and brings out their worst reactions. They need to replace animosity and narrowness with generosity and intelligence. And that's the purpose of the workshop in this chapter.

Yes, it's a Catholic workshop, and to some that means another kind of narrowness. Can a Catholic workshop really encourage young people to think for themselves? Doesn't the church expect us to look for mindless compliance with official teachings?

The workshop in this chapter will be Catholic in a much larger and truer sense. In an age of educated believers, when Catholics have learned to be thinkers in every other area of their lives, the renewed church of Vatican Council II no longer seeks to teach by rote indoctrination:

> The search for truth . . . must be carried out in a manner that is appropriate to the dignity of the human person . . . , namely by free enquiry with the help of teaching or instruction. . . . It is by personal assent that [people] must adhere to the truth they have discovered. (*Declaration on Religious Liberty*, no. 3)

The renewed church of Vatican Council II teaches about faith and morality no less vigorously or authoritatively than before. Like any great teacher, the church speaks with a certain urgency to persuade, and even warn, believers about what is true and wholesome. But now, at the same time, our church wisely extends an attitude of profound respect for the process of inquiry and discovery by which people arrive at sound beliefs and values.

This Catholic workshop, then, will ask all participants to become thoroughly engaged in Catholic teaching on homosexuality. The young people will be asked to respect the wisdom and authority of the church's voice enough to test its teaching with their own questions, ideas, and concerns. In short, young people should meet the magisterium as thinkers seeking to understand, not as robots ready to be programmed.

Such truth work is holy, for it allows the Holy Spirit, also called the "Spirit of Truth" (John 16:13), to move and work. For it is only by the Spirit's work that our mind really opens and the light of truth actually dawns. Our job is to create the right conditions for the Spirit's work.

If the Spirit of Truth is to succeed in this workshop, another very powerful spirit—the spirit of violence—must first be renounced by all participants—youth and adult.

All disdainful attitudes and antagonisms against homosexuals, against the church, against one's own feelings, and against ministries of support and healing must be left outside the door of the workshop. Otherwise the discussion will not be safe. Expressions of mindless disrespect can quickly poison the atmosphere of openness and trust on which this workshop depends.

No class or youth group should simply be led into this workshop by its teacher or adult leaders without prior discussion and an agreement to create together a climate of strong mutual respect. The whole session preceding the workshop must be devoted to seeking this mutual understanding and commitment to respect. Otherwise the workshop should not happen.

Is the group willing to commit in advance to a nonviolent exploration of such a violence-laden issue, willing to differ but not divide, to disagree but not disrespect? Are the participants willing to create together an experience of church in which all are free to think and explore and open their minds to truth?

(Permission to reproduce this introduction is granted.)

Discussion In leading discussion of the following questions, please keep in mind that the subject of the first session is not homosexuality but the various forms of violence that surround homosexuality and therefore make it impossible to discuss peacefully. When comments about homosexuality itself come up—and they probably will—just gently defer them to the next session and refocus on the question at hand.

In brackets, I have supplied possible answers to the following questions. These answers can be added to those the young people provide.

1. What antihomosexual attitudes have you seen in your school or in the news?
   [A gay sailor in the U.S. Navy was brutally beaten to death by one of his shipmates.]
2. What anti-Catholic expressions have you heard or read regarding the church's teaching on homosexuality or any other controversial issues?
   [Gay activists disrupted Mass at Saint Patrick's Cathedral in New York City by scattering condoms on the altar.]
3. What effects do you think fear of homosexuality has on young people?
   [Young people may destroy their own natural affection for same-sex friends.]
4. In your opinion, why are the testimonies of people who have been freed of homosexuality by Christian support and healing ministries routinely discredited by the media?

[The media are afraid that any evidence indicating that homosexuality is not natural and permanent will justify antihomosexual attitudes.]

5. What pitfalls do we, as a group, have to be careful to avoid in order to explore safely the issue of homosexuality?
[The participants need to avoid talking as if gays or lesbians are "out there" somewhere, because some of their fellow group members may feel that they are gay or lesbian.]

6. Is everyone ready to commit to total mutual respect in a discussion of the subject of homosexuality?
[Pay careful attention to any no answers and pursue them with the group until the dissenters are all satisfied.]

Finally, ask the members of the group to phrase their commitment to one another in a single sentence that can be read at the start of session 2 for the benefit of anyone who missed session 1.

Session 2	## Participants' Workshop
Introducing the Workshop	**Opening Comments**

Opening Comments
The leader begins the workshop by asking a young person to read the commitment to mutual respect that the group formulated at the end of session 1. The leader then comments on that commitment:

> This agreement is the golden key that can unlock a workshop that will be helpful to everyone. The agreement will allow you to express your ideas about homosexuality without fear of antagonism from one another. It will leave you free to think new thoughts and find new wisdom on an issue that most people only argue about.

> Someone may have second thoughts about this commitment, or someone who missed session 1 may have come to this session, so ask the young people again: Is everyone here willing to make this commitment of mutual respect to one another?

Passages and Prayers
A peer leader then reads the following two scriptural verses, which capture the workshop tone that everyone has agreed to seek: "'Do not judge, so that you may not be judged'" (Matt. 7:1, NRSV). "'When the Spirit of truth comes, he will guide you into all the truth'" (John 16:13, NRSV).

A second peer leader then offers the following prayer, reading slowly and deliberately, so that the Spirit can work in every heart while the prayer is being read:

O God, please forgive us. We are a violent nation. Please forgive us especially for any violence of thought, word, or deed any of us has committed against our gay brothers or lesbian sisters—any insult or injury, any prejudice or slander. Please rid our society, our church, and our hearts of temptations to such violence. Please grant us instead the courage to give love, to listen, to be honest, and to be a friend.

Lord Jesus, please free us from any antagonism toward the church that this issue may have caused us. Please release into our workshop your Spirit of Truth so that on this issue of such confusion and hurt, we can be open to the church as we seek your caring response to people you send into our life who are facing homosexuality. Please prepare us to be their friends and to help them find your path of love for them.

Lord, we are all searching and growing in our sexuality. Please keep us free from fear as we listen to our heart and to your gentle and guiding Holy Spirit, so that we will always have the courage to trust you and to love, no matter where our path may lead. Amen.

Ground Rule
The adult leader repeats a final ground rule for the workshop— the one that was emphasized in session 1:

Please remember that what you express tonight will personally affect anyone here who is dealing with homosexual feelings. And guess what? Sooner or later that may include many of us. The word from the field of psychology is that a significant percentage of people experience homosexual feelings at some time during adolescence.

The attitude we shape tonight will not only affect everyone here but also people we will meet and befriend in the future—people who will need to know our feelings on the subject. In fact, the workshop is especially designed with them in mind.

So let our focus be love—not our ego, not who's right. It's fine to disagree, but let's do so in order to seek further truth, not to win an argument. Let's wrestle with this issue so as to push one another deeper into love's wisdom. That way everybody wins. Fair enough?

Workshop Steps

Before beginning step 1 of the workshop, a peer leader hands out a stapled set of resources to all the participants. These resources are provided at the end of this chapter. The set of resources includes the following:

4–A "Friendship Survey"
4–B "First Friendship Response"
4–C "Second Friendship Response"
4–D "Organizations That Serve Homosexuals"
4–E "The Voice of the Church and the Scriptures"
4–F "The Voices of Contemporary Psychology"
4–G "The Voices of Science"
4–H "A Letter to My Friend"

Step 1: Presenting the Issue

The purpose of the first step is not to resolve anything, but rather, to let everyone feel the significance of the issue for their own life and to see the importance of developing sound values about it.

The leader presents the issue in the following manner:

> First of all, why is it so important for all of you to work out your values on the subject of homosexuality, which directly affects only a minority of the population? There are two good reasons: one that affects your relationship with your family and friends, and the other that affects your relationship with the church.

Family and friends: The leader continues the presentation of the issue with the following words:

> It is safe to say that at some point someone close to you, maybe a friend or a family member, will come to you and confide that he or she is dealing with homosexual feelings or behavior. What will you say? Will you stay close or back away? Will you encourage or discourage the person's homosexual feelings or behavior? Perhaps you haven't yet encountered that situation or had that conversation, but it's safe to say you will. Our society is becoming more and more open about homosexuality, and people are beginning to talk about their sexual orientation with those who are close to them.

Next, to help the group grasp the importance of thinking through this issue and clarifying their values regarding it, the leader asks the young people to write their responses to the following questions from part A of resource 4–A, "Friendship Survey":

1. Are you acquainted with someone who is homosexual, that is, gay or lesbian?
2. Has anyone ever confided in you about her or his homosexual feelings or experiences?
3. How might you react to someone who confided in you about their homosexuality?
   - Would you back away?
   - Would you give assurances of unchanged friendship?
   - Would you feel that you were rejecting the friend if you did not give your approval of her or his homosexual choices?
   - Would you give your approval?
4. If your friend decided to enter into homosexual activity, would you question that decision?

At this point the leader gives the participants the following instruction:

> Put a star beside whichever one of your answers is most significant to you. [They take a moment to do this.] Any of you who feels comfortable doing so is invited to share your most significant answer with the group—not for discussion, just to make us all aware of one another's responses.

The church: The leader now continues the presentation of the issue with the following:

> The issue of homosexuality is also important to each of us because our church upholds a position that many people in the United States do not support.
>
> A great debate is raging in society about homosexuality. In 1986, the Vatican reaffirmed its position that homosexuality is an "objective disorder," and that being a homosexual person is not sinful, but homosexual activity is morally wrong ("The Pastoral Care of Homosexual Persons," no. 3). Noting also "enormous pressure . . . on the church . . . to condone homosexual activity," the 1986 Vatican document calls that point of view "profoundly opposed to the teaching of the church" (no. 8).
>
> The American Psychiatric Association (APA), on the other hand, voted in 1973 to remove homosexuality from its official list of disorders. It was a close vote, strongly influenced by an intense lobbying effort by the gay movement. It should also be noted that many psychia-

trists who voted against that decision still offer treatment for recovery from homosexuality as a disorder, while others regard even the concept of a "cure" for homosexuality as offensive. (David Gelman et al., "Born or Bred," *Newsweek* [24 February 1992]: 49)

If you are Catholic, those differing views leave you caught right in the middle—especially when someone grappling with homosexuality comes to you for support. What can you say that won't either offend your friend or ignore your church?

To illustrate the religious and moral tensions we face with this issue, the leader asks the group to write their responses to the following questions from part B of resource 4–A:
1. Are you troubled or reassured by the church's and the Bible's disapproval of homosexual activity?
2. Do you believe that homosexual activity is just as healthy for some people as heterosexual activity is for others?
3. Do you believe that homosexual activity is unhealthy for those who have homosexual inclinations?
4. Do you feel that you have understood this issue well enough to take a firm stand on it? [This last question can also be asked of the group as a whole, with the response being in the form of a show of hands.]
Again invite the participants to put a star next to their most significant answer and then share it with the group. But don't discuss the answers.

After the participants have finished sharing, the leader continues the presentation of the issue in the following manner:

> I propose to you that the issue of homosexuality is important enough to warrant all of us opening our preconceived positions. We need to help one another think about what is the most loving and Christian response to a homosexual person. And we must clarify for ourselves values that support that response.

Step 2: Exploring Two Responses to Confiding Friends
First, the leader explains that the purpose of step 2 is to consider potential responses to homosexual persons and the possible consequences of those responses.

Next, the leader describes the format of step 2 in the following way:

We will now consider two responses that you might have to a friend who confides in you about her or his homosexual tendencies.

The question that we will use to focus our discussion remains the same all the way through the workshop: What do you say to a friend who is trying to come to terms with homosexual feelings and tendencies?

Let's assume you are not just going to walk away from your friend, and your friend knows that. Let's also assume that your friend really wants you to be honest and say what you think. In a real situation, of course, the friend may not want to hear what you think. In that case, there's probably no need to go into your values about homosexuality. And if not, then don't. But for the purposes of this workshop, the scenario is that you are being asked sincerely, as a Catholic friend, what you believe. You are on the spot. What do you say?

Resources 4–B and 4–C present two responses a person in your shoes might make.

The leader instructs the participants to read silently resource 4–B, "First Friendship Response," which is located at the end of this chapter.

When the participants have read the first response, the leader asks them to come up with possible consequences of this response. Then the leader lists these consequences on a chalkboard or a sheet of newsprint. If the young people have a hard time coming up with possible consequences, the leader offers any of the following to get them started:

- Your friend might feel greatly relieved about your continued friendship and your attitude of inquiry about homosexuality.
- Your friend might already feel scared or discouraged by his or her homosexuality and may feel great comfort that you are searching. As a result, your friend may find the courage to begin searching too.
- Your friend may feel rejected by God because the church regards him or her as having a disorder, as not being like God intended human beings to be. If so, you will need to talk a lot about how God loves us just as we are.
- Your friend may have been tempted to turn off God or the church because of the stance that some members take, and your response may make him or her feel included again.
- Your friend might be glad to hear about other gay and lesbian believers who stay Catholic.

When all the consequences of the first response have been listed, the leader asks the group to read resource 4–C, "Second Friendship Response."

After the participants have read resource 4–C, the leader again asks them to list the possible consequences of such a response. If they have a hard time coming up with possible consequences, the leader mentions a couple of these to get them started:

- Your friend might be looking for support for her or his homosexual tendencies and for that reason may get mad and call you bigoted or homophobic. She or he may even stop being your friend.
- Your friend might be looking for support for her or his homosexual tendencies, but even though you don't support them, she or he may "agree to disagree" about them and keep a firm grip on the friendship you have.
- Your friend might feel troubled about her or his homosexual tendencies, and it may be of great help just to talk about what has been going on.
- Your friend might feel troubled about her or his homosexual tendencies and want them to stop. If so, she or he may want to learn about other resources that can be of help.

The leader next notes that the responses make references to two organizations—Courage and Exodus International. Courage expresses the Catholic church's approach of supporting people who are dealing with a homosexual orientation. Exodus International is an ecumenical network of many ministries from many Christian churches, all of which agree fully with the Catholic church's teaching on homosexuality. Both organizations have local chapters across the country to support people who are dealing with a homosexual orientation. The leader points out that resource 4–D presents descriptions of these organizations.

Step 3: Listening to the Voices of the Church and the Scriptures, Psychology, and Science
Step 3 expands the discussion by letting in some new voices. The goal is that by listening to the church and the Scriptures, psychology, and science, the young people will gain insights and values that will help them respond to a homosexual friend.

The message of each voice can be quickly grasped using this method with resources 4–E, 4–F, and 4–G:

- Introduce each resource with the points provided in the leader introduction.

- Have the participants read the resources silently.
- Ask for volunteers to summarize for the group what each voice has to say. Make sure that important points are not omitted.
- Add your own comments, using the leader commentary as a guide.

It is crucial in this step to restrict discussion and stick to the sole purpose of getting out the information.

Background for the leader on the voice of the church and the Scriptures: The goal of resource 4–E is to familiarize the participants with church teaching about homosexuality by having them read excerpts from an actual church document. The participants should gain a grasp not only of what the church says, but of how deeply the church cares for homosexual people.

Leader's introduction: The leader introduces resource 4–E with these words:

In speaking about any of a wide range of faith or morality issues—homosexuality being only one such issue—the church functions in the role of teacher. The church in its teaching role is called the *magisterium*. Like any good teacher, the church speaks as persuasively as possible in an effort to influence and guide its listeners. The church speaks from much love, long experience, deep conviction—and something more.

Catholic Tradition holds that the church has the responsibility, handed down from Christ and directed by the Holy Spirit, to teach from a posture of reliable authority on matters of faith and morals. When teaching in the role of magisterium (from the Latin word for "master"), the church is regarded as expressing the teaching voice of Christ himself.

That's a startling claim with which we Americans, who especially value our independence of thought, certainly have to struggle. However, Catholic Tradition does not demand of us mindless agreement with the magisterium. Rather, church Tradition demands the kind of honest, respectful, and vigorous dialog on the issue that we would bring to Christ himself. In that spirit, you are invited to read the material on resource 4–E.

(I also recommend the new *Catechism of the Catholic Church*, which contains another clear, concise, and usable expression of the church's teaching on homosexuality. As we go to press, the official English translation is not yet available.)

The participants are directed to read silently resource 4–E, and then they are invited to summarize for one another, but not to discuss, the contents of that reading.

Leader's commentary: The leader makes these comments about the church's teaching on homosexuality:

> Many times over the two thousand years since Christ established the church as his voice on earth, that voice has challenged the prevailing ideas of a culture. Ours is one of those times, and we are one of those cultures that the church is now challenging.
>
> A prophet's voice often meets with strong resistance, but that's the church's job—to be the conscience of a culture—just as it is the job of our conscience to challenge us.
>
> The church's teaching on homosexuality is challenging and unpopular, but no one who reads it can claim that is unloving, although many who have not read it make that claim. And many Catholics who do not know the teaching are embarrassed and caught off guard by that claim.
>
> As you think about church teachings and develop your conscience on the complex subject of homosexuality, you can be assured of one fundamental thing: Your church stands firmly on the side of love.

Background for the leader on the voices of contemporary psychology: The goal of resource 4–F is to help the participants understand the majority view of the field of psychology about homosexuality—a view that disagrees with the church's teaching—in a way that allows them to keep their respect for the church's teaching and for the discipline of psychology.

Leader's introduction: The leader introduces resource 4–F with these words:

> The church and the field of psychology work together in great harmony and mutual respect on most issues, because both share a great commitment to the well-being and happiness of every individual. But that commitment has led to opposing views on the issue of homosexuality.
>
> Psychology and the church are institutions that are greatly trusted in society, so the disagreement on homosexuality is difficult for us as Roman Catholics. We would

certainly prefer to place our total trust in the wisdom of both the church and psychology. However, because that is not possible, careful and respectful thinking is needed in order to find an understanding that interprets this disagreement in a way that leaves intact our positive regard for both institutions—because we need them both.

One key difference can help clarify why the church and psychology come to such different conclusions about homosexuality—they have different starting points. The church always bases its thinking on God—on what God has done in creation and has spoken through prophetic individuals over the church's long history. Harmony with God and God's creation, the church believes, is the secret to human happiness.

Psychology, on the other hand, does not think in God terms. Some psychologists may, but they do so on their own. Officially, psychology thinks strictly in human terms. That's its strength and its weakness too. Psychology maintains that the feelings and goals of the individual are paramount and that harmony with self is the secret to human happiness.

Most often, these two approaches and disciplines, when they are conducted responsibly, do not conflict. But on this issue, where God's purposes for sex are so central to the church's thinking and so absent from psychology's view, the two institutions do come to opposite conclusions. You are invited to read the material on handout 4–F with this difference in mind.

The participants are directed to read silently resource 4–F, and then they are invited to summarize for one another, but not to discuss, the contents of that reading.

Leader's commentary: Next, the leader offers the following comments:

On a number of sexual issues besides homosexuality, the church takes a strong moral stand, and psychology does not. Again the difference is that psychology does not share in the church's conviction about the God-given sacredness of marriage and procreation. That list of issues includes premarital sex, marital fidelity, artificial birth control, and abortion. And for non-Christian cultures, that list would include such practices as polygamy, infanticide, and ritual sex. The discipline of psychology does not claim for itself the right to make moral judgment on such matters.

The church insists that true human happiness, which is the common goal of church teaching and psychology, must include a moral perspective that goes beyond the immediate inclinations of the person. The church also dares to speak, because that is its prophetic responsibility to humanity, about what values will be best for a whole culture.

Background for the leader on the voices of science: The goal of resource 4–G is to introduce the debate about the origins of homosexuality as being just that—a genuine scientific debate, not (as many people have been led to believe) an issue that science has already resolved. Thus when the news media report research findings as if science has ended all debate and proven conclusively that all homosexuality is natural and normal, our young people will be aware of the moral and political agenda driving that research and that reporting.

Leader's introduction: The leader introduces resource 4–G with these words:

Much of the controversy in the world of psychology swirls around the issue of whether some people are actually homosexual by way of physical makeup. That's a big unsettled question. Psychologists who report success in curing the homosexual condition say it has it origins in early emotional damage, which can be reversed.

On the other hand, the official majority viewpoint of psychology bases its treatment approach on the assumption that at least some people are born homosexual. That's a big assumption. Solid answers to this question must be pursued beyond the realm of psychology.

And answers also must be pursued beyond the realm of the church. The magisterium actually remains neutral on this question of the origin of homosexuality, but in the world of science, the question is being hotly debated. And the debate is being conducted in the appropriate realm of science, which is research. You are invited to read resource 4–G and listen to the voices of science as they report and debate their conflicting findings.

The participants are directed to read silently resource 4–G, and then they are invited to summarize for one another, but not to discuss, the contents of that reading.

Leader's commentary: The leader offers the following comments about resource 4–G:

Research findings about the origins of homosexuality appear frequently in the news. Those findings tend to be reported as if the debate is now over and homosexuality has been proven to be natural and not a disorder at all. That conclusion, of course, makes the church's teaching seem out of touch with the latest discoveries of modern science. Science actually is still far from making such a final conclusion. The media's premature conclusion reflects their well-intentioned political and moral bias; they are working hard to reduce antihomosexual hatred by establishing acceptance of homosexuality in the public mind. While the church shares and supports the news media's responsible desire to lessen antihomosexual attitudes, the church also teaches that much more than unquestioned acceptance of homosexuality is entailed in truly loving homosexual people.

Step 4: Formulating a Response

Step 4 has two parts. In the first part the participants are invited to formulate for themselves a list of caring and thoughtful points they would want to make in response to a friend who had confided in them about her or his homosexual feelings or experiences. The young people are to draw these points from all the discussion and evidence they have heard and read. In the second part they are asked to incorporate the points into a letter of response that they would be willing to send to their friend. After giving an overview of this activity, the leader sets the tone for it with the following words:

> The church invites you to listen carefully to church teaching and then challenges you to exercise your God-given freedom to choose the highest possible values for yourself and to form the clearest possible conscience for yourself. That freedom carries with it an awesome responsibility. Your values and choices determine the shape of your moral life and physical lifestyle. Even beyond your own life, your ideas profoundly influence the life of people who trust you. That's how important these points and letters are. Please pray as you work.

To begin, the leader asks everyone to write down on resource 4–H a preliminary list of points they would want to include in their response to their friend.

Then the leader divides the group into small groups. The participants combine their individual lists into a single list of points that their small group would include in a letter of response.

Next, each small group writes its list of points on newsprint, complete with dissenting opinions, and presents it to the large group.

When I conducted this activity with my group, much agreement and disagreement emerged in our list. However, a number of points did surface that everyone agreed were essential to responding to a friend who is dealing with homosexual feelings or experiences. Here are those points:

1. I accept the person and reaffirm our friendship.
2. I want a mutual honesty that will not threaten our relationship.
3. I want to try to hear and feel whatever my friend has gone through.
4. I encourage my friend to maintain a prayer life and a sacramental life.
5. I urge my friend to resist self-labeling and to leave room for possible emotional changes.
6. I encourage my friend to surrender his or her thinking and choices about homosexuality to Christ and to ask for his light.

The values reflected in those six points of agreement represented a group consensus and a rather passionate commitment to the friend.

Beyond those six points of agreement, individuals expressed widely diverging opinions for or against the positions of the voices presented to them in the workshop. That divergence of opinion, rather than being viewed as a problem to be resolved, was regarded as necessary to the intent of the workshop. That intent was to allow honest disagreement to be expressed in an atmosphere of goodwill and genuine inquiry.

To complete step 4, all the participants, in the quiet of their own conscience, composed a letter to their friend expressing how they felt now, after having thought about the issue all the way through the workshop.

Closure

At this point in our workshop the room was filled with unanimous goodwill, even though the opinions were far from unanimous. We ended the workshop with a prayer similar in form to the prayers of the faithful, but the intentions for our prayer came spontaneously from the group. We found that this kind of prayer provided a suitable and unifying conclusion to the workshop.

Post-Workshop Reflections

1. The workshop was discussion dynamite. Even young people who were typically quiet had much to say. The workshop profoundly stretched them to think with a new breadth of love. It stirred their best passions and gave them a place to express their thoughts and feelings about this issue.

2. Most young people in our group came to the workshop having been strongly influenced by the gay movement as presented to them through the media or their school. By and large they came with the impression that all people with homosexual feelings and attractions have felt that way since birth. Accordingly, they thought that the way to deal with homosexuality in all cases was to accept it.

3. The young people also thought that happiness for a homosexual had to include physical sexual expression. It was new to them to learn of homosexual people who are not at all in conflict with the church but, in fact, enjoy the full support of the church and are living happy lives of abstinence from sexual activity.

4. Also new to the participants was the fact that some persons who had regarded themselves as homosexual since birth, but were not able or willing to accept their orientation, found it possible to make a transition to heterosexuality.

5. We found that the role of the church as teacher on any issue was not well known to our young people. For them, mother church was a remote sort of parent, a would-be Vatican teacher who was not well bonded with her children. When a controversial issue such as homosexuality came along, the church was easily written off. We had referred to church teachings on other occasions, but just referring to them clearly had not made enough of an impact. This was the first time we had studied material directly from the church documents. Such careful listening to church teaching was a new experience for the group. They did not know that Catholic Tradition views the teaching voice of Christ himself as being expressed in the wisdom of the magisterium.

6. A crucial element of the workshop was the unconditional love that was directed toward anonymous group members who were struggling with homosexual tendencies regardless of whether their personal hopes were to enter the gay lifestyle successfully, to find help in becoming free from homosexual tendencies, or to regard their homosexual inclinations as a passing adolescent phase.

7. For the sake of another secret problem some members of the workshop might be carrying, here is a statement I now include just before the closing prayer. You might want to include something like it.

> In most groups of young people, some members have been sexually abused by someone of the same or other sex. If that is you, your experience has probably been on your mind throughout the workshop. You need to know something that you may have a hard time believing: What happened is not your fault, and it does not make you a bad person. And there is one more thing I want you to hear and take to heart: I would be deeply honored if you ever want to talk to me about that experience and let me help you figure out how to put it completely behind you.

If you make this invitation you will probably get some takers—perhaps not right at the moment, but later. When that time comes, your job will be to listen with all your heart. And after you have been entrusted with the story, ask the young person if just sharing it with you is relief enough or if he or she would like to talk further with a counselor who could help even more. But even if the young person does not pursue the matter further, do not underestimate what you have provided by just listening.

We adult leaders, acting on behalf of the church, did model to our young people one distinct value that some may find controversial—the value of their continued search for wisdom on the subject of homosexuality. That value was unanimously welcomed, and in return, the young people granted to the church careful and respectful attention to Catholic teachings. The group did not offer unquestioning compliance, but rather deep concentration with the church on finding the way of truth and love. Here is how Saint Paul regarded the unfinished work of formation in people whose conversion he influenced: "I am quite confident that the One who began a good work in you will go on completing it until the Day of Jesus Christ comes" (Phil. 1:6, NJB).

We might never know the views on homosexuality that our workshop participants will eventually develop. Yet we rest assured that they will arrive at consciences based on deep listening to the church, vigorous thought, great compassion, and intense prayer. Could we ask for more?

Friendship Survey

Write your responses to the following questions on a separate sheet of paper.

Part A

1. Are you acquainted with someone who is homosexual, that is, gay or lesbian?
2. Has anyone ever confided in you about her or his homosexual feelings or experiences?
3. How might you react to someone who confided in you about their homosexuality?
   - Would you back away?
   - Would you give assurances of unchanged friendship?
   - Would you feel that you were rejecting the friend if you did not give your approval of her or his homosexual choices?
   - Would you give your approval?
4. If your friend decided to enter into homosexual activity, would you question that decision?

Part B

1. Are you troubled or reassured by the church's and the Bible's disapproval of homosexual activity?
2. Do you believe that homosexual activity is just as healthy for some people as heterosexual activity is for others?
3. Do you believe that homosexual activity is unhealthy for those who have homosexual inclinations?
4. Do you feel that you have understood this issue well enough to take a firm stand on it?

Resource 4–A: Permission to reproduce this resource is granted.

First Friendship Response

You're amazing. You know better than anyone that my Catholic faith is important to me, and you had no idea how I would react, but you took the leap anyway.

My reaction may surprise you. I've also really needed to talk with someone about homosexuality. My struggle has not been about homosexual feelings, like yours. Rather, mine has been about beliefs. I truly believe Christ speaks to the world through the church's teachings, and now I'm hearing a lot of people say that the church is old-fashioned and just plain wrong about homosexuality.

I feel caught in the middle and torn apart. So you're really doing me a big favor by being so honest. Your love crisis and my faith crisis are really similar, so let's go through them together. Maybe we can help each other.

I've always been incredibly proud that my church, in its teachings and in its actions, stands up for peace and for poor people. I know church teachings are the voice of Christ, because they are the voice of love. But I'm not one to live my life and think my thoughts only inside the church. The church recognizes that it can learn much from voices in the secular world, such as the voices of science, democracy, and psychology. But in this case, the voice of the world and the voice of church teaching are deadlocked about what you are going through.

Church teaching says homosexuality is a disorder. Psychologists used to say that, but they officially reversed themselves and now claim homosexuality can be healthy. The media are full of stories about gay rights and gay-bashing. The church did stand up for gay rights when the state of Oregon had a referendum to take them away, and the referendum was defeated. However, the gay movement says that's not enough, that it is also a violation of rights not to support homosexual lovemaking.

Church teaching maintains that it is not wrong to have homosexual feelings, but homosexual activity is morally wrong. A movement of Catholics, called Dignity, claims that the church is wrong and needs to change because homosexual preferences are God-given. The church teaches that groups like Dignity are misguided and dangerous.

Okay, I take seriously what the church teaches, and it hurts me when people attack the church over its stance on homosexuality. Yet my faith cannot be a blind faith either. I need to understand how telling you not to have homosexual contact can represent Christ's love for you.

I do understand church teachings in other areas. For instance, the church teaches that any time we forget that the sex act is a bonding, reproductive act meant for married couples and carry it outside of marriage, we get ourselves in trouble—in the teen pregnancy rate, the abortion rate, and many other areas. But how does a homosexual love life do damage?

I guess the church is teaching that you'll be hurting yourself if you enter a homosexual lifestyle. Maybe that's true in some way we can't grasp yet. All I can say to you is I'm confused right along side you. I do know your long-term happiness is on the line here, so for your sake and my own, I can promise you I'm going to keep listening, thinking, and praying about this issue until I really do understand it.

Second Friendship Response

Thank you for telling me what's been happening. If you hadn't, our friendship would have suffered. You showed a lot of courage in your honesty, and I'm going to try to match it.

So what do I think—especially being Catholic? First, I think it's just crazy to be having sex of any kind at our age. I know a lot of people do, but just look at how many people are getting badly hurt.

Second, can you say for sure that you're homosexual? Almost everyone our age at some point has some sort of homosexual feelings or desires. You could easily get yourself locked into a gay or lesbian lifestyle by labeling yourself at this time and by not giving yourself a chance to keep growing and changing.

So that's my advice. It's pretty close to the church's teaching about homosexuality: It's not your fault. You can't help the way you feel, just don't act on it. I've always had one problem with that advice. It always seemed to me almost cruel for God to create homosexual people and then say, "Don't act on those feelings." So I did some checking around for other options and found some interesting things.

Did you ever hear of Courage? It's a church-supported movement for homosexual people who don't believe in the gay or lesbian lifestyle. Courage offers support groups that treat homosexual tendencies as addictions. Courage operates like other twelve-step recovery groups.

Many people in Courage, if they want more than just self-control—I mean if they really don't want their homosexual orientation—are being referred to another kind of ministry that helps them awaken heterosexual feelings through healing therapy and prayer.

Those programs are part of a movement called Exodus International, which has ministries in many Christian denominations (including Catholic) and has helped a lot of people make the journey out of homosexual orientation. You're probably wondering if such a journey is even possible. You may be thinking: Aren't some people just born homosexual, just like some people are born black or white? Maybe so, I don't know. There's a lot of debate about that in the scientific world, and the church takes no position on either side.

I do know that Exodus reports a high success rate, and not just with people who only feel partially homosexual. Many ex-gays (as they call themselves) say they had never had even the slightest twinge of heterosexual impulse their whole life. They had always felt they were different—permanently. All that changed for them when they learned to let in love, support, and especially prayer to touch long-standing insecurities about their masculinity or femininity stemming from early childhood. They say their stalled sexual selves just started to grow again.

Well, that's what I found out, and I think it's pretty hopeful. Maybe it sounds good to you; maybe it doesn't. But please don't think my friendship for you depends on what you decide to do. We've both taken a risk here by being honest, and I don't want to lose our friendship over this issue. If we disagree, let's just agree to disagree and still be good friends, okay?

Organizations That Serve Homosexuals

Courage

Courage was founded in 1980, and it supports homosexual Catholics who accept the church teaching that sexual physical expression between homosexuals is not in accord with Catholic Christian morality. Members of Courage use the twelve-step method developed by Alcoholics Anonymous to seek support and spiritual strength for abstaining from physical sexual expression of their homosexuality. Courage emphasizes fellowship, inner peace, spiritual growth, and a close relationship with Christ. Recently, Courage has begun to inform its members of therapies and ministries that can help those who desire a heterosexual orientation.

The Courage brochure states, "Courage is a spiritual support group for Catholic men and women—and their families—who are striving to live chaste lives in accordance with the Catholic Church's teaching on homosexuality."

Courage has approximately twenty chapters in the United States and three in Canada. The national office is in New York City.

Exodus International

Exodus International is an ecumenical organization that was founded in 1976 to bring together spiritual and therapeutic ministries that help men and women who believe that their homosexual orientation can change and who want to change it. The Exodus approach focuses the healing power of Christ and same-sex peer support on old hurts and fears that may have prompted a homosexual orientation. Many of the Exodus board members and leaders are people who formerly practiced a homosexual lifestyle but went through a recovery process that gave them confidence in their own masculinity or femininity and a gradual emergence of their response to the other sex.

The Exodus brochure describes itself as "an umbrella organization" that provides an annual conference and a communication and referral service for ministries that enable the male or female homosexual to "shed the old identity." The Exodus approach is consistent with Catholic teaching.

Exodus maintains a referral list of about sixty-five support groups and ministries in thirty-three states, as well as two in Canada. The national office is in San Rafael, California.

Resource 4–D: Permission to reproduce this resource is granted.

71

The Voice of the Church and the Scriptures

The Voice of the Church

The following quotations are from a 1986 Vatican letter entitled "The Pastoral Care of Homosexual Persons":

> The church, obedient to the Lord who founded her and gave her the sacramental life, celebrates the divine plan of the loving and life-giving union of men and women in the sacrament of marriage. It is only in the marital relationship that the use of the sexual faculty can be morally good. A person engaging in homosexual behavior therefore acts immorally. (No. 7)

> To choose someone of the same sex for one's sexual activity is to annul [erase] the rich symbolism and meaning, not to mention the goals, of the Creator's sexual design. Homosexual activity is not a complementary union able to transmit life. (No. 7)

> Although the particular inclination of the homosexual person is not a sin, it is a more or less strong tendency ordered toward an intrinsic moral evil and thus the inclination itself must be seen as an objective disorder. (No. 3)

> Therefore special concern and pastoral attention should be directed toward those who have this condition, lest they be led to believe that the living out of this orientation in homosexual activity is a morally acceptable option. It is not. (No. 3)

> This does not mean that homosexual persons are not often generous and giving of themselves. (No. 7)

> It is deplorable that homosexual persons have been and are the object of violent malice in speech or in action. Such treatment deserves condemnation from the church's pastors wherever it occurs. It reveals a kind of disregard which endangers the most fundamental principles of a healthy society. The intrinsic dignity of each person must always be respected in word, in action, and in law. (No. 10)

> Increasing numbers of people today, even within the church, are bringing enormous pressure to bear on the church to accept the homosexual condition as though it were not disordered and to condone homosexual activity. (No. 8)

> The church's ministers must ensure that homosexual persons in their care will not be misled by this point of view, so profoundly opposed to the teaching of the church. (No. 8)

> No authentic pastoral program will include organizations in which homosexual persons associate with each other without clearly stating that homosexual activity is immoral. (No. 15)

> We would heartily encourage programs where these dangers are avoided. (No. 15)

The homosexual orientation in certain cases is not the result of deliberate choice. (No. 11)

In fact, circumstances may exist or may have existed in the past which would remove or reduce the culpability [fault] of the individual in a given instance; or other circumstances may increase it. What is at all costs to be avoided is the unfounded and demeaning assumption that the sexual behavior of homosexual persons is always and totally compulsive [unable to stop one's self] and therefore inculpable. (No. 11)

What is essential is that the fundamental liberty which characterizes the human person and gives him his dignity be recognized as belonging to the homosexual person as well. As in every conversion from evil, the abandonment of homosexual activity will require a profound collaboration of the individual with God's liberating grace. (No. 11)

One dissident Catholic organization stands out as the object of the cautions in the Vatican document quoted above. Dignity, founded in 1973, teaches, in opposition to the magisterium, that gay and lesbian lifestyles and sexual expression are "consonant with Christ's teachings." The church opposes organizations like Dignity in very strong terms, calling them "misleading" and "dangerous."

The Voice of the Scriptures

The Scriptures say this about homosexuality: "'You shall not lie with a male as with a woman; such a thing is an abomination'" (Leviticus 18:22, NAB).

In a listing of sexual impurities, Paul includes these: "females exchanged natural relations for unnatural, and the males likewise gave up natural relations with females and burned with lust for one another" (Romans 1:26–27, NAB).

The Voices of Contemporary Psychology

Psychology as a respected voice in society is new. Most people trace its beginnings to the work of Sigmund Freud early in the twentieth century. Freud regarded homosexuality as a psychological disorder. That was the shared understanding for the first sixty years of the new mental health movement. Then, in 1973, that majority view reversed itself when the American Psychiatric Association (APA) voted by a close margin to remove homosexuality from its official directory of disorders.

So psychology has a new majority position, but a majority is not a consensus. For that reason, this presentation of what psychology has to say about homosexuality must be carefully dated and must also present the climate of great controversy, incomplete research, and political struggle that still surround the subject.

The following summary is based on my conversations with a variety of psychotherapists on both sides of the homosexuality question:

There is an informal consensus among a current majority of therapists that a small percentage of people are exclusively homosexual and a small percentage are exclusively heterosexual. Everyone else falls in between, with varying degrees of homosexual and heterosexual tendencies.

People in the middle range might sometimes be confused about their sexual orientation, especially during adolescence when sexuality is normally in transition. Many adolescents experience homosexual feelings and desires, and some even experiment with homosexual activity. This experimentation does not necessarily indicate an exclusive homosexual condition, even when it leads to gay or lesbian relationships.

For the purposes of counseling about homosexuality, contemporary psychology operates on the assumption that people in the middle range do have a choice about their sexual orientation and the lifestyle they lead. However, the small percentage of people who find themselves exclusively attracted to the same sex are regarded as being homosexual from birth. These persons are counseled to accept the sexual orientation they have and to ask the same acceptance of people around them.

Therapy includes much encouragement from the counselor about the wholesomeness and naturalness of homosexual feelings. An effort is made to counteract any inner attitudes picked up from family, friends, society, or religion that would suggest that the homosexual orientation is a disorder or that homosexual physical expression is wrong.

The decision of the APA to stop calling homosexuality a disorder is often explained to the homosexual person. And such a client is encouraged to seek support beyond counseling sessions by "coming out" to friends and loved ones, seeking their support for his or her emerging confidence as a gay or lesbian person as well for his or her present or future gay or lesbian relationships.

The "coming out" process is difficult and requires a lot of courage, because so many inner and outer antihomosexual feelings must be overcome in developing this new confidence. In the context of that struggle, reports of treatment plans that cure homosexuality are seen as sources of confusion and as barriers to the process of establishing a firm homosexual identity.

Not surprisingly, most therapists who foster that process of homosexual identity affirmation respond very negatively to colleagues whose approach is to help clients control and overcome rather than affirm their homosexual orientation. Both camps, though motivated entirely by goodwill, often see each other as enormously destructive in their impact on clients.

Both camps claim to relieve the severe depression that often accompanies homosexuality, especially among adolescents—no doubt they both do. The political struggle that ensues from these conflicting viewpoints within the world of psychology is intense.

The majority view among therapists is challenged by an organization called the National Association for Research and Treatment of Homosexuality (NARTH). NARTH therapists publish articles and hold conventions on research and treatment approaches that aim for recovery from homosexuality. The work and even the ethical principles of these therapists are frequently attacked by their peers. But it should be noted that the church's call to abstain from homosexual behavior is consistent with NARTH's treatment approach.

The Voices of Science

The voices of science are voices of current research that is at the cutting edge of what we know about the biological origins of homosexuality.

A well-known and well-loved passage sets the tone for an openness to what science has to say about homosexuality: "'You shall know the truth, and the truth will set you free'" (John 8:32, NAB).

Listen now to a pair of truth-seeking voices from science, each of them testing out one of two main hypotheses about the origins of homosexuality. One of them is trying to determine whether homosexuals are "born that way," the other is trying to determine whether homosexuals are "formed that way" in their families.

The genetic hypothesis: Simon LeVay, a neuroscientist at the Salk Institute in La Jolla, California, has evidence to support his theory that homosexuality is genetic. His findings were reported in the 24 February 1992 issue of *Newsweek* magazine. LeVay scanned the brains of forty-one male cadavers, including nineteen homosexuals, and discovered that the hypothalamus, a tiny part of the brain believed to control sexual activity, was less than half the size in the gay men than in the heterosexuals. This may be the first "direct evidence of what some gays have long contended— that whether or not they choose to be different, they are born different" (Gelman et al., "Born or Bred," page 46).

Newsweek critiqued LeVay's discovery by offering a second finding reported by another scientist at the Salk Institute: "A body of evidence [shows] that the brain's neural networks reconfigure themselves in response to certain experiences. One fascinating NIH [National Institutes of Health] study found that in people reading Braille after becoming blind, the area of the brain controlling the reading finger grew larger" (Gelman et al., "Born or Bred," page 50).

Newsweek also reported findings from a study at Northwestern University stating that "if one identical twin is gay, the other is almost three times more likely to be gay than if the twins are fraternal—suggesting that something in the identical twins' shared genetic makeup affected their sexual orientation" (pages 46, 48). But critics of the study wonder: If genetics is the determining factor, why do so many identical twins have opposite sexual orientations? (page 52).

The environmental hypothesis: A second hypothesis is that of Joseph Nicolosi, a clinical psychologist and director at the Thomas Aquinas Psychological Clinic in Encino, California. Nicolosi's evidence supports a familial (formed that way) theory of homosexuality. His findings were also reported in the 24 February 1992 issue of *Newsweek* and in the 20 October 1991 issue of the *National Catholic Register*. Nicolosi has treated over 165 Catholic and actively homosexual men who sought therapy because their religious values did not match their gay lifestyle. About 90 percent of those clients developed heterosexual responsiveness, suggesting that in those cases, homosexuality was a treatable disorder and not genetic.

Nicolosi, whose program is part of the Exodus network, employs an approach he calls gender-deficit group therapy. His approach strives to strengthen a homosexual male's masculine identity so as to overcome the need to look for it in another male. This method combines strongly supportive masculine bonding and an uncovering of old defenses and hurts to allow in the warmth of the group energy and to let it heal the hidden selves of members. Deep comfort with masculinity then develops, and along with it spontaneously comes interest in the other sex. Many therapists associated with Exodus International have used a similar approach to help lesbian women.

In April 1992, Nicolosi was interviewed on "20/20" with a recently married, happy former client. Then a second psychologist came on to say that he had treated several clients who previously had become heterosexual through a similar kind of therapy and had come to him deciding to revert back to homosexuality.

So nothing is conclusive, and the search for truth goes on. Regarding the question of both the origin and the treatment of homosexuality, church teaching takes no position.

The scientists conducting research on the origins and treatment of homosexuality may not be impartial truth-seekers. Some are motivated by passionate and political concerns about the impact of their research on human lives. That's not to say their passionate commitment is something negative, but it calls for a certain caution from us as news consumers. As new research findings are reported in the media, we should read those articles with an awareness of the political and even religious agenda and biases of the researchers and the the news organizations reporting that research.

A Letter to My Friend

1. List points that express what you would want to convey to a friend who has confided in you about homosexual feelings or experiences.

When all the small groups have shared their list of points, add to your list any points that you feel you left out.

2. Write a letter to the person you have been imagining throughout this workshop. Express the kind of support you feel will be most helpful.